Essential Oils:

350+ Essential Oils Recipes, Tips, References, & Resources - Aromatherapy Homemade Natural Remedies to Improve Your Health & Skin, Lose Weight, Overcome Anxiety, Stress & Depression!

Kevin Moore © 2016

All rights reserved. No part of this book may be reproduced in any form without permission in writing from the author. Reviewers may quote brief passages in reviews.

Disclaimer:

This book is for informational purposes only and the author, his agents, heirs, and assignees do not accept any responsibilities for any liabilities, actual or alleged, resulting from the use of this information.

This report is not "professional advice." The author encourages the reader to seek advice from a professional where any reasonably prudent person would do so. While every reasonable attempt has been made to verify the information contained in this eBook, the author and his affiliates cannot assume any responsibility for errors, inaccuracies or omissions, including omissions in transmission or reproduction.

Any references to people, events, organizations, or business entities are for educational and illustrative purposes only, and no intent to falsely characterize, recommend, disparage, or injure is intended or should be so construed. Any results stated or implied are consistent with general results, but this means results can and will vary. The author, his agents, and assigns, make no promises or guarantees, stated or implied. Individual results will vary and this work is supplied strictly on an "at your own risk" basis.

Introduction

First off, thanks for purchasing my book "Essential Oils: 350+ Essential Oils Recipes, Tips, References, & Resources - Aromatherapy Homemade Natural Remedies to Improve Your Health & Skin, Lose Weight, Overcome Anxiety, Stress & Depression!" By grabbing this book you've shown that you're interested in learning about all the wonderful possibilities afforded to us when using essential oils in our daily lives.

This book will teach you what you need to know to get started using essential oils. I'll be discussing the different types of essential oils and all of their amazing benefits. I'll also be going over a ton of easy to create essential oil recipes and the different ways they can be used to improve your life. I hope you fall in love with essential oils the same way I have over the years. It's had an incredibly positive impact on the lives of my family and I know it can have one on yours if you let it.

During the course of this book, I'll be going over all the tools and resources I use. I've also included answers to many of the frequently asked questions I hear from those new to the world of essential oils. If you're familiar with essential oils, I hope you enjoy all the recipes I've included. They should keep you busy for the foreseeable future. However, you don't need any prior experience with essential oils in order for this book to benefit you.

I'm excited to begin. Let's get started!

Chapter One: An Introduction To Essential Oils

An Introduction To Essential Oils

So what are essential oils? Well, an essential oil is a type of liquid that is normally distilled (usually by water or steam) from stems, leaves, bark, flowers, roots and other elements of a plant. Even though referred to as an oil, they do not give off an oily feeling. Many essential oils are actually clear, while some like orange, patchouli, and lemongrass are yellow or amber in color.

Essential oils are so wonderful because they contain the pure essence of the plant it's derived from. Since essential oils come highly concentrated, a tiny bit will go a long way. Many people confuse essential oils with fragrance oils or perfume. They are not the same. While essential oils are derived from the actual plant, perfumes and fragrance oils are created artificially and therefore may contain artificial ingredients. Perfumes and fragrance oils do not contain any of the therapeutic benefits associated with essential oils.

The aroma and chemical composition of essential oils can provide physical therapeutic benefits along with valuable psychological benefits. These benefits are normally achieved through the application of the oil to your skin or by inhalation.

Essential oils have been around for thousands of years. Many cultures have you used them to treat and alleviate illnesses throughout history. Every major civilization from the ancient Egyptians onward has harnessed the power of essential oils to improve the life of its people. Essential oils were so important that two of the three gifts said to be given to Jesus were myrrh and frankincense, both forms of powerful essential oils.

Many essential oils are often used by diluting them using a carrier oil and then applying the blend to your skin for absorption. A few examples of carrier oils are apricot kernel oil, sweet almond oil, and grapeseed oil.

Carefully inhaling certain essential oils can also have a therapeutic benefit. As oil molecules enter into the lungs they get absorbed into your bloodstream.

Essential oils normally get sold in tiny individual bottles. They can vary a great deal in both price and quality. Some of the factors that will affect the price and quality of your oil will include the plant's rarity, the standards of the people distilling the oil, the country and climate where the oil comes from, and how much oil get produced per plant.

When purchasing essential oils you can get either individual oils or blends of several oils. The advantage of purchasing blends is that it can save you time and money having to buy each individual oil and mixing them. The main disadvantage is that since you're not mixing it personally, you have no control over the blend and you can't reliably mix the blend you've purchased with any other oils.

What Are Absolutes?

Absolutes are very aromatic liquids that are extracted from plants. Absolutes, however, get extracted in a highly complex manner that includes the use of chemical solvents that then get removed later during the last stages of being produced. Sometimes a small trace amount of the chemical solvent may remain in the final product.

Although this trace amount of solvent is considered very small in extracted absolutes, essential oils that are steam distilled are preferred by practitioners of holistic aromatherapy. That being said, absolutes are still used, one just needs to do so with respect, care, and knowledge. In general, absolutes are not ingested internally due to the trace amounts of solvent they may contain.

Essential Oils Extraction Process

Essential oils are extracted from nature using a few different processes that I will discuss in this section.

Distillation

The majority of essential oils are obtained through this process. Raw plant materials such as roots, seeds, fruit peels, woods, and leaves are placed inside a distillation device. The water in the device containing the plant parts is then heated and the steam is passed through the device eventually vaporizing all the volatile compounds which are collected in a receiving vessel. This process will normally take several hours from start to finish. Some essential oils obtained using this process include lemon, lavender, and clary sage.

There are different forms of distillation from the one I mentioned above. Some of these are water distillation, steam distillation, and hydro-diffusion.

Expression

This process involves obtaining the essential oil through mechanical extraction. It is often referred to as cold pressing. The process was more popular before distillation was invented. It involves getting the essential oil from citrus peels. This method works on citrus essential oils only and was often done by hand. The peels contain a good amount of essential oil in them.

First, the peel or rind would be soaked in warm water, then a sponge would be used to press on the peel or rind. This would break up the protective layer of the peel and soak up the essential oil. Once that was completed, the sponge would be pressed over some form of container to collect the essential oil. Once pressed into the container, it would be left to stand so the oil had time to separate from the juice water. The final step would then involve siphoning the essential oil from the container. More modern methods of expression include the use of centrifuges and other modern machinery.

Solvent Extraction

This process involves extracting essential oils from plant parts containing small amounts of oil. For example, extracting essential oils from flowers is notoriously difficult due to the small amount of essential oil they contain. Therefore a solvent, such as hexane, is used to get the essential oil. These finished products are also referred to as absolutes, which I discussed in the last section.

Methods of Using Essential Oil

Adding essential oils to your life can be fun, easy, and beneficial to your health. In this section, I'll be going over some of the ways you can get started. Each of these different methods provide their own set of benefits and safety concerns. Always be sure to follow all applicable safety precautions and pay attention to how certain oils are to be used or not used in specific situations. Don't forget that essential oils are powerful and therefore need to be used with some caution. It's also important to keep in mind that essential oils are also flammable so keep them away from open flames or sparks.

Aromatherapy Massage

Add the amount of essential oil called for in your recipe to your carrier oil and massage the mixture on your partner or yourself. Always be sure to keep these blends away from your genitals, eyes, and mouth. Never apply essential oils directly to your skin without diluting the oil first. Always be sure to read any safety information on the oils you end up using.

Bath

Add the amount of essential oil called for in your recipe to your carrier oil. Mix it together and add your blend to your running water in the bath. Be sure to mix it again before entering the tub. Always be sure to read any safety information on the oils you end up using.

General Household Cleaning

Add the amount of essential oil called for in your recipe to your wash, trash can, drain, laundry, tissue, or vacuum bag filter. There are a million ways to incorporate essential oils into your household on a daily basis. Always be sure to read any safety information on the oils you end up using.

Insect Repellent

Add the amount of essential oil called for in your recipe to your cotton balls or tissues and place them near your windows and doors to repel any insects. There are a ton of wonderful oils that act as repellent for insects. These include peppermint, lavender, and my personal favorite citronella. During the summer, when I'm having guests over, I have posts surrounding my yard which I use citronella oil on. This helps to repel any insects from bothering us. Always be sure to read any safety information on the essential oils you end up using.

Pet Care

Add the amount of essential oil called for in your recipe to your carrier oil. Apply to your pets as laid out in the directions of whatever recipe you're using. Always be sure to read any safety information on the oils you end up using. Be very careful when using essential oils on your pets. I recommend not trying this until you've gained some experience working with them.

Room Freshening

Add the amount of essential oil called for in your recipe to 2 cups of boiling water that's been placed in a bowl. Don't inhale into the bowl, instead, let the steam carry the oil throughout the room. Some people use this method, while many stick to scent rings or diffusers. I personally have a diffuser in every room of my home. Always be sure to read any safety information on the oils you end up using.

Simple Inhalation

Place approximately 3 to 4 drops of your essential oil on your tissue. Place your tissue near your nose area and deeply inhale. When first trying out an oil, only use a single drop to ensure that you're not sensitive or allergic to that type of essential oil. Always be sure to read any safety information on the oils you end up using.

Steam Inhalation

Boil 2 cups of water. Pour your water into your bowl and add approximately 3 to 7 drops of essential oil to your water. You may want to consider using fewer drops if you're dealing with an oil that can cause irritation to your mucous membranes. For example, cinnamon, rosemary, thyme eucalyptus, and pine.

Place your nose approximately 12 inches away from your bowl and deeply inhale. Be sure not to inhale the steam on a constant basis. If you start to feel any kind of discomfort, stop right away. Steam inhalation is great for dealing with influenza and colds. Use of relaxing or energizing essential oils can also make this particular method useful. Keep your eyes closed when inhaling the steam. Always be sure to read any safety information on the oils you end up using.

Other Uses

Besides the methods listed above, essential oils can be made into facial toners, lotions, soaps, perfumes, shampoos, and other types of natural products. Essential oils are extremely versatile in the ways they can be used to benefit us in our daily lives. In this book alone I go over more than 350 essential oil recipes you can use to help benefit you, your pets, or your home.

What is Aromatherapy?

Aromatherapy is, in essence, the practice of using different varieties of volatile plant oils, including essential oils, for our physical, spiritual, emotional, and mental well-being.

In addition to using essential oils, aromatherapy also encourages the use of other types of complementary naturally found ingredients including hydrosol, sugars, sea salts, clay, herbs, milk powders, mud, cold pressed vegetable oils, and jojoba (a type of liquid wax).

Aromatherapy frowns up the use of any kind of synthetic ingredients being used. Always be careful when purchasing products that are marketed with the word aromatherapy on their labeling or packaging. This word is not regulated in the US and many products out there on the market contain ingredients that are synthetic. These products should be avoided. That's why it's always important to read the labels before you buy.

The same can be said for items labeled essential oils or natural ingredients. Those labels can be misleading and may contain synthetic ingredients along with the oils or natural ingredients they are claiming to be made with. Good sellers should always be happy to provide you with a list of the ingredients in their essential oils or other products. That's why I suggest only purchasing your essential oils and supplies through reputable companies. In the resource section, I give a bunch of reputable places I use to purchase my essential oils.

Inhaling Essential Oils Benefits

Essential oils that are inhaled into your lungs can offer both physical and psychological benefits. The aroma of your essential oil stimulates your brain to trigger a specific reaction, but when it is inhaled into your lungs, the natural constituents can supply a wonderful therapeutic benefit. For example, diffusing eucalyptus oil can help you ease congestion. Always be sure to use your essential oils correctly. Not doing so could have serious repercussions and side effects.

Topical Application Essential Oils Benefits

Essential oils that are topically applied to your skin get absorbed into your bloodstream. The constituents of an essential oil can aid in areas like beauty, health, and hygiene. Since essential oils are incredibly concentrated and powerful, they shouldn't be applied topically to your skin in their undiluted form.

To apply an essential oil to your skin, one should dilute the essential oil using a carrier oil. A few examples of carrier oils include grapeseed oil, sweet almond oil, and apricot kernel oil. I'll touch on a few more different kinds of carrier oil in the next chapter.

Other Essential Oil Benefits

In addition to the emotional, spiritual, mental, and therapeutic benefits of essential oils, they can be used in a variety of other applications. Essential oils can be used in natural pesticides and insect repellent, household cleaners, and pet care.

Essential Oil Blends

A big upside of essential oils is that they can be mixed and matched to form new complex blends and aromas. In a later chapter, I'll go over 350+ recipes you can make on your own for a variety of different applications. Oftentimes, essential oils that are blended together can have a greater effect than if you had them working independently.

You should always be careful when blending together essential oils. When you're first starting out I would steer clear of any of the oils I mention as hazardous in the next chapter. I would also hold off on using them around children, pets, or pregnant women until you have much more experience working with them. It's always a good idea to find a good aromatherapist in your area and have them help you with any blends or recipes that can cause serious side effects if done improperly.

Types of Diffusers

I will often get asked what kinds of diffusers are best and what are the differences between the different types of diffusers. Unfortunately, there's no one right answer to this question. A lot of this comes down to personal preference or the specific situation you're using the diffuser for. In this section, I'll discuss the four different categories of available diffusers. Each type of these diffusers puts your essential oils into the air. Each one has its own set of benefits to consider. I use everything but heat diffusers. I don't like to heat up my essential oils but that's just a personal preference.

Evaporative Diffusers

These diffusers are pretty simplistic in the way they operate. You have a fan that blows air from your room through a filter or pad that contains essential oils dropped on it. The air that is blowing through your pad causes your oils to evaporate at a quicker rate than normally, while the air containing your evaporated oil is being blown into your room.

This type of diffuser is ideal for getting your oil scent into your room. However, due to the way it evaporates you don't get the whole essential oil all at once. Instead, you get the lighter components in the oil at the start of the process and the heavier components near the end of the process. What this means is that the therapeutic properties of the oil may be diminished thereby lessening the effects.

Overall, this is a good form of diffusion that quietly diffuses your aroma throughout an entire room. They make a wide variety of these diffusers. Everything from battery operated versions to diffuser jewelry versions which you can wear.

Heat Diffusers

These are similar to the evaporative diffusers, however, they use heat instead of air blowing to accomplish the diffusion. While some types of heat diffusers will use a higher level of heat to produce a stronger smell, the top heat diffusers only use a lower level of heat to produce a more subtle and subdued aroma. The level of heat you're using is very important. The higher the heat the more you can alter the chemical properties of your essential oils.

These types of diffusers share the same issues as the evaporative diffusers. They don't get the whole essential oil at once. The good thing about these diffusers is they are completely silent and cost effective to use. They do a good job of putting your oil's aroma into your room.

Nebulizing Diffusers

A nebulizer basically works in the same fashion a perfume atomizer does. A small jet of air blowing across a small-sized tube creates a type of vacuum that actually pulls your liquid at the bottom of your tube up to the top of your tube. The air that is flowing across the surface of your oil at the top of your tube blows your oil away in a mist or fine spray. When used with a consistent air supply source, this kind of diffusion will put a lot of oil in the air quickly.

Since this kind of diffusion is working to put your whole oil out into the air in tiny droplet form, it's often thought to be the best kind of diffusion for the therapeutic use of your essential oils. Since these nebulizing diffusers are working to quickly saturate the air with your essential oil, they will normally run at a higher level of sound and will also use your essential oil at a much higher rate than the other kinds of diffusers. When using these diffusers it's a good idea to run them on a timer so that there only running for approximately 15 minutes every hour. This will allow you to conserve your essential oil and cut down on your costs. It will also allow your olfactory system some time to process the oils that you've received and allow you to recover before getting more.

Ultrasonic / Humidifying Diffusers

Similar to nebulizing diffusers, ultrasonic diffusers will also create a fine mist. However, the method it uses to accomplish this is very different. With an ultrasonic diffuser your utilizing different electronic frequencies to make a small-sized disk under the surface of a liquid, like water, to begin vibrating at an extremely fast rate. These ultrasonic vibrations will then break your essential oils down into tiny micro-sized particles, dispersing your oil in the form of a fine mist. These smaller particles are much more easily absorbed by your lungs for a better therapeutic effect on your mind, spirit, and body.

While transforming water or liquids into a vapor will normally require a lot of heat, the transformation of your liquids into a vapor occurs through an adiabatic process. This means the means the liquids changed states without using any type of heat energy.

This kind of diffusion will make a nice mist that will humidify the air and gives off the sound of water trickling, although only a tiny amount of your mist is actually your essential oil and it will depend completely on the room's air current to actually disperse your mist through the entire room. This makes this type of diffuser ideal for people who only want a small amount of essential oil to be diffused into their room.

Reasons To Use Essential Oils

Essential oils are so popular because they offer solutions to so many different problems people face in their day to day lives. This versatility is virtually unmatched by any other set of products I can think of. In this section, I'm going to go over some of the many reasons one can use essential oils.

Aches, Pains, & Common Ailments

Essential oils are wonderful for treating everything from minor aches and pulled muscles, to sores, cuts, and burns. If there's something wrong with your body there's more than likely a combination of essential oils that can help ease your discomfort and quicken the healing process.

Cleaning Products

If you don't want to clean your home using products filled with harmful chemicals then you're going to love all the cleaning recipes I've included later on in this book. I try and use as many of these as I can in my own home. Not only are they a healthier alternative to store bout solutions they're also effective. It's hard to beat a combination like that.

Colds, Flu & Congestion

Don't like taking pills and other forms of doctor prescribed medication? Want something natural to help you get rid of that cold or your cough? If so, then you'll want to check out some of the recipes I have that focus in treating colds, flu, & congestion using a variety of essential oils. I also include recipes to help boost your immune system so you never fall ill in the first place.

Emotional Support & Mental Clarity

Essential oils are often used to help treat conditions like depression. Essential oils can stimulate the limbic system in our brain. They can be used for all different types of emotional issues ranging from anger and abandonment issues to grief, worthlessness, and fear of failure. Essential oils are also great for helping us focus and achieve mental clarity. Back in college, I used to use essential oils whenever I had to study for an exam. I'm naturally unfocused, meaning I could always use the extra boost my essential oils provided me with.

Love & Relationships

Looking for love in your life? Want to attract someone? Aroma plays a big part in who we desire and who we don't. I've included a few aphrodisiacs to help you find that special someone in your life.

Mood & Energy

Not only can essential oils keep us relaxed they can also be used to give us a shot of much-needed energy. Not only that but certain essential oils can directly affect a person's mood and outlook on life. I love using my oils whenever I'm feeling a little down or lazier than usual. I find they do an excellent job of lifting my spirits and getting my engine going. I've included many of my favorite recipes in a later chapter of this book.

Pet Care

Essential oils can be great for your pets. I've included a bunch of different recipes you can use to help improve the life of your pet. I suggest not trying these on your pets before you've got some experience handling essential oils. Personally, I waited a long time before ever using an essential oil on them. I tend to err on the side of caution but the safety of my pet is always my utmost concern.

Relaxation

Essential oils are excellent for helping one center themselves and find a deeper sense of peace and relaxation. Different recipes and aromas have a way of triggering our mind to slow down and remove any anxiety or stress that may be negatively affecting us.

Room Freshener

Essential oils can be used to make your home smell fresh and inviting. I've included a bunch of recipes perfect for all types of occasions and seasons.

Skin & Hair Care

Essential oils can treat everything from a mild case of acne to a severe form of eczema. Essential oils can also protect your lips, hands, feet, and hair. In a later chapter, I'll be going over a bunch of different recipes to combat all forms of skin and hair care issues. Not only can essential oils help cure existing issues it can also help prevent issues in the future. It will make your skin and hair healthier than ever before.

Weight Loss

If you want to drop a few pounds then essential oils like grapefruit oil, ginger oil, and cinnamon oil will aid you in the process. I've included recipes for everything from cellulite removers and appetite suppressors to metabolism boosters and weight loss remedies.

Chapter Two: Types of Carrier Oils & Essential Oils

Types of Carrier Oils

In this section, I'm going to go over a list of common carrier oils, what they do, and some of the different types. This will give you a good reference for later on when you're trying to determine what oils to use for the purpose your trying to achieve.

Carrier oils are a necessity if you plan on using your essential oils for anything besides cleaning products. A carrier oil is just a liquid form of vegetable oil that is used to help dilute the highly concentrated essential oil you want to use.

Here are a list of my favorite carrier oils and a little bit about each one.

Borage Seed Oil

This is a good choice when trying to treat a skin condition such as acne. It is also known for its anti-inflammatory properties and is good for combating gout, clotting disorders, and arthritis. This oil should be avoided by people with liver conditions and by women who are pregnant.

Coconut Oil

Great for moisturizing the lips, hair, and skin. Has lubricating properties which make it an ideal choice for massage. This carrier oil is a little more difficult to handle than some of the others as it remains a solid when at room temperature. Has a very fragrant aroma and is highly stable with an oily feel to it. I don't mess with this type of oil too often as I'm not a fan of the aroma.

Fractionated Coconut Oil

This type of oil is simply coconut oil that's had the longer chain fatty acids removed from it. The difference between this and regular coconut oil is that it stays liquid when at room temperature, making it much easier to handle and use in applications with essential oil. It's a very stable oil with a long shelf life and it's affordable which makes it a nice option if you're on a budget.

People who prefer all natural oils will want to stay away from this as it has been tampered with chemically to remove some of its natural compounds. This oil is naturally colorless and odorless. It also doesn't have a greasy feeling which is something I appreciate.

Jojoba Oil

I use this in a lot of the recipes you'll find later in this book. I find it to be an extremely useful carrier oil and one of my favorite choices. This type of carrier oil is really a wax. It's incredibly stable to use and comes with a longer shelf life. This type of oil acts like a natural anti-inflammatory and is great for inflamed skin or in the use of massage. This type of oil is suited for people who are prone to acne and have oily skin. This carrier oil absorbs nicely and has a distinct smell that I quite enjoy.

Marula Oil

This is a great oil known for its antioxidant properties. It's easy to work with and highly stable. Does a good job of both hydrating and healing your skin at the same time. This type of oil is harvested from the nut located inside the Marula fruit located in Africa. This is a wonderful oil for skincare, hair, and beauty regimens in general.

Sweet Almond Oil

My personal favorite carrier oil. This is an excellent all-purpose oil. It's inexpensive to purchase and has a shelf life of around 1 year. This type of oil absorbs quickly while leaving only a hint of oil on the skin. I use this oil in a bunch of recipes later on in this book. This is a one you'll want to have on hand.

Types of Essential Oils

In this section, I'm going to go over a list of common essential oils and what they are known for. This will give you a good reference for later on when you're trying to determine what types of essential oils to use for the purpose you're trying to achieve.

Angelica Root Oil

This type of essential oil has a peppery and woody aroma to it. This oil is known to stimulate one's immune system, fight off infection, and eliminate toxins. This oil has often been used in combating anxiety, stress, and different forms of exhaustion. This oil is intense and is often blended with other oils instead of being used solely on its own. It has a very distinctive woodsy and peppery aroma to it.

This is a phototoxic oil and once applied should not be directly in any type of UV light. Could cause blistering and irritation to the skin if it's exposed.

Anise Oil

This type of essential oil has a rich licorice aroma to it. This oil reminds me of black licorice, something I'm not personally a fan of. This is a powerful essential oil known for its use in treating many types of ailments such as colds, flu, congestion, muscle aches, coughing, and flatulence. This type of oil is also said to stimulate menstruation and increase the production of breast milk.

This oil should be avoided in pregnant women and children under the age of 5.

Basil Oil

This type of essential oil has a sweet licorice aroma to it. This is a great oil to use when needing to focus or stimulate your mind. It has many antiviral and antibacterial properties which make it ideal when feeling under the weather with a cold. This type of oil is also popular for treating flatulence, exhaustion, gout, flu, insect bites, and coughs.

Should preferably be used only during the morning hours and daytime hours. This type of oil should only be used sparingly.

Bay Oil

This type of essential oil has a spicy, fruity, medicinal aroma to it. This a warming oil that is perfect for the fall and winter months. This oil is ideal for helping heal muscle pulls and muscle strains. It's also known for stimulating circulation. Other reasons for using this oil include the treatment of dandruff, treating oily skin, and hair care.

This oil can inhibit blood clotting so always be careful to use the amount recommended.

Bay Laurel Oil

This type of essential oil has a fresh and fruity aroma to it. Different from regular bay oil this oil is great for emotional support and promoting a higher level of courage and confidence. This oil is known as a good expectorant and therefore is ideal for use in certain diffuser blends, especially those combating illness such as colds and flu. Other reasons for using this oil include the treatment of poor appetite and tonsillitis.

This oil can lead to a higher rate of issues when applied topically. Use extra care when applying this oil on your skin. Make sure it's always correctly diluted. Never place on skin that is damaged.

Bergamot Oil

This type of essential oil has a citrus and floral aroma to it. This oil is known for increasing one's energy and boosting one's mood. It has an amazing complex citrus infused aroma that is a personal favorite of mine. This oil is great for treating grief, halitosis, cold sores, depression, stress, acne, loss of appetite, itching, and oily skin.

This type of oil is extremely phototoxic and therefore once applied proper precautions must be made to avoid all UVA rays. This includes tanning beds and direct sunlight on the area treated topically for a period of 24 hours.

Black Pepper Oil

This type of essential oil has a fresh, crisp, peppercorn aroma to it. This isn't an oil I use often. It's good for improving arthritis, increasing alertness, easing sore muscles, improving digestion, relieving constipation, and increasing stamina. This oil should be avoided at night time as it's liable to keep you up past your bedtime.

This is a relatively safe and stable oil. No real precautions except not to misuse or abuse as are the case with all essential oils.

Caraway Seed Oil

This type of essential oil has a sweet, spicy, and fruity aroma to it. This oil is used more in fragrance blends than holistic ones. When used holistically it is often a part of blends, especially those that are geared towards men. It's a good expectorant that is sometimes used in diffuser blends to help combat bronchitis and colds. This type of oil is also used as an energy booster and as a way to ease coughing and the effects of laryngitis.

This is a relatively safe and stable oil. No real precautions except not to misuse or abuse as are the case with all essential oils.

Cardamom Oil

This type of essential oil has a rich and woody aroma to it. This is a great oil for both therapeutic and aromatic blending. This is a very popular blending oil as it goes well with many other types of essential oils. It's known as a good expectorant that is used to help relieve stress, depression, and fatigue. It's also used to help combat a loss of appetite, halitosis, and colic.

This type of oil should be avoided by younger children, especially around their face. Can cause breathing problems and CNS.

Carrot Seed Oil

This type of essential has a warm, earthy, and woody aroma to it. This oil is used primarily in skin care regimens. It's known for helping with damaged and mature skin. This oil is not generally used in aromatics due to its unpleasant aroma. It's more geared towards helping with issues like gout, water retention, eczema, and removal of toxins.

This type of oil should be avoided during both breastfeeding and pregnancy.

Cassia Oil

This type of essential oil has a spicy cinnamon aroma to it. This oil is used primarily in fragrance blends. It has an aroma similar to that of cinnamon oil. It's also known for helping with relieving gas, diarrhea, indigestion, rheumatism, colic, and colds.

This type of oil should be avoided by younger children and pregnant or breastfeeding women. Can cause blood clotting issues. It can also cause irritation to the skin when applied topically. Be very careful when using this oil. Do not use more than is called for in a recipe.

Catnip Oil

This type of essential oil has a herb and mint aroma to it. This oil is used often as an insect repellent. This oil is generally used as an anesthetic, sedative, astringent, anti-rheumatic, and anti-inflammatory.

This oil can cause irritation to the skin when applied topically. Be very careful when using this oil. Do not use more than is called for in a recipe.

Cedarwood Oil

This type of essential oil has a sharp, woody, and sweet aroma to it. This oil has been popular since the ancient Egyptians. It's known for it's calming and grounding properties. This oil is generally used to combat negativity, arthritis, stress, dermatitis, coughing, dandruff, bronchitis, and as an aphrodisiac. This is a popular oil in masculine blends.

This is a relatively safe and stable oil. No real precautions except not to misuse or abuse as are the case with all essential oils.

Cinnamon Leaf & Bark Oil

This type of essential oil has a rich cinnamon aroma to it. Cinnamon leaf oil is usually less well received than cinnamon bark oil but is a cheaper alternative. These oils are often used to treat low blood pressure, flatulence, stress, constipation, scabies, lice, exhaustion, regulating blood sugar levels, reducing inflammation, rheumatism, and improving insulin sensitivity.

These types of oil can cause skin irritation and mucous membrane irritation. They should be avoided by both children and women who are pregnant or breastfeeding. Be very careful when using these oils. Do not use more than is called for in a recipe.

Citronella Oil

This type of essential oil has a nice fresh, sweet, citrus aroma to it. This oil is generally used to help fight against headaches, fatigue, oily skin, and excessive perspiration. It is also a popular insect repellent and one of my favorite ways to ward off bugs in the summertime.

This is a relatively safe and stable oil. No real precautions except not to misuse or abuse as are the case with all essential oils.

Clary Sage Oil

This type of essential oil has a bright and earthy aroma to it. I often use this in my diffuser blends. This oil is generally used to help deal with a sore throat, gas, exhaustion, stress, asthma, labor pains, and coughing.

Studies suggest one should avoid consuming alcohol when using this type of essential oil. Women with breast cancer or at higher risk for breast cancer should also steer clear of using this essential oil.

Clove Bud Oil

This type of essential oil is known for it's spicy and woody aroma. This oil is often used to deal with sprains, strains, arthritis, toothaches, rheumatism, and bronchitis.

This type of oil can cause skin irritation and mucous membrane irritation. It can also inhibit blood clotting and should be avoided by younger children.

Coriander Oil

Sometimes referred to as cilantro oil. This type of essential oil has a sweet, spicy, woody aroma to it. It is normally used to relieve the effects of arthritis, fatigue, colic, nausea, indigestion, rheumatism, and general aches.

This is a relatively safe and stable oil. No real precautions except not to misuse or abuse as are the case with all essential oils.

Cumin Oil

This type of essential oil has an earthy and spicy aroma to it. This oil is normally used to relieve the effects of bad circulation, low blood pressure, fatigue, gas, indigestion, stomach cramps, colic, and relief from a toxic build up in our system.

This essential oil should be avoided by women during pregnancy.

Cypress Oil

This type of essential oil has a woody evergreen aroma to it. It's excellent to use in blends with other oils. It really helps with concentration and alertness. This oil is also used to combat hemorrhoids, oily skin, rheumatism, and excessive perspiration.

This is a relatively safe and stable oil. No real precautions except not to misuse or abuse as are the case with all essential oils.

Eucalyptus Globulus Oil

This type of essential oil has a fresh strong earthy aroma to it. It's great for dealing with the flu, fever, arthritis, poor circulation, coughing, cold sores, bronchitis, and colds.

This oil should not be used around young children, especially near their faces as it can cause breathing issues and CNS. This essential oil should not be ingested as it can be toxic when taken internally.

Fennel Oil

This type of essential oil has a sweet and earthy aroma to it. It's excellent for helping to improve digestion, reduce weight gain, achieve more peaceful sleep, and suppress appetite. It's also good for healing bruises, flatulence, nausea, and halitosis.

This essential oil can inhibit blood clotting and may react poorly with medication. Women who are pregnant or breastfeeding should not use this oil.

Fir Needle Oil

This type of essential oil has a woody sweet fresh aroma to it. This oil is perfect for fighting coughs, colds, flu, bronchitis, sinusitis, rheumatism, and muscle aches.

This essential oil can cause skin irritation, especially if oxidized. Be careful when applying topically.

Frankincense Oil

This type of essential oil has been popular since biblical times. Has a fruity and spicy aroma to it. This oil is great for fighting anxiety, stress, scars, coughing fits, stretch marks, and bronchitis.

This essential oil can cause skin irritation, especially if oxidized. Be careful when applying topically.

Geranium Oil

This type of essential oil has a fresh and sweet aroma to it. This oil is perfect for dealing with lice, acne, oily skin, menopause, and dull skin.

This essential oil can have adverse reactions when taken with some types of medication. If you're on medication always check for any drug interactions before using this oil.

German Chamomile Oil

This type of essential oil has a sweet and fruity aroma to it. This oil is ideal for dealing with arthritis, allergies, boils, flatulence, dermatitis, insomnia, strains, sprains, wounds, PMS, earaches, cuts, insect bites, inflamed skin, and headaches.

This essential oil may have a negative reaction when used with certain medication. If taking medication be sure to check any drug interactions before using.

Ginger Oil

This type of essential oil has a warm and spicy aroma to it. It's great for improving circulation and is a popular oil in blends for massage. This oil is ideal for fighting motion sickness and nausea. This oil is a good mood booster and is perfect for people with arthritis and muscle aches.

This essential oil is very powerful and should be used carefully. This oil has low levels of phototoxicity. Be sure to avoid sunlight and other UV rays after applying topically.

Grapefruit Oil

This type of essential oil has an uplifting, crisp, and sweet aroma to it. This oil is wonderful for curbing cravings, boosting metabolism, increasing endurance and energy, reducing abdominal fat, reducing water retention, and dealing with dull skin. This oil also makes a great disinfectant and antiseptic. One of my most used essential oils.

This essential oil is highly phototoxic. Be sure to avoid sunlight and other UV rays after applying topically.

Helichrysum Oil

This type of essential oil has a fresh and earthy aroma to it. This is oil is ideal for boils, acne, cuts, wounds, eczema, skin irritation, dermatitis, and burns.

This is a relatively safe and stable oil. No real precautions except not to misuse or abuse as are the case with all essential oils.

Hyssop Oil

This type of essential oil has a fruity, woody, and slightly sweet aroma to it. This oil is great for dealing with sore throats, coughing, and bruising. I use this one quite often when feeling under the weather.

This essential oil should be avoided by both children and by women who are pregnant or breastfeeding. Be very careful when using these oils. Do not use more than is called for in a recipe.

Juniper Berry Oil

This type of essential oil has been popular since ancient times. This oil has a crisp, sweet, and earthy aroma to it. This oil is great for dealing with gout, acne, colds, rheumatism, obesity, and lowering the amount of toxins in the body. This oil is a natural antiseptic and can provide emotional support when diffused or burned as incense. Another one of my favorite essential oils.

This is a relatively safe and stable oil. No real precautions except not to misuse or abuse as are the case with all essential oils.

Lavender Oil

The essential oil I use most often in my day to day life. This type of essential oil has a fresh, floral, sweet aroma to it. This oil is ideal for dealing with anxiety, allergies, stress, strains, sprains, vertigo, insect bites, headaches, asthma, earaches, bruises, burns, oily skin, hypertension, labor pains, sores, and rheumatism. This is a must have essential oil and one of the first ones you should be purchasing when starting out.

This is a relatively safe and stable oil. No real precautions except not to misuse or abuse as are the case with all essential oils.

Lemon Oil

This type of essential oil has a clean slightly sour lemon aroma to it. This oil is ideal for increasing energy levels, enhancing mood, relieving pain, suppressing weight gain, improving dull and oily skin, curing athlete's foot, and getting rid of varicose veins.

This essential oil is phototoxic when cold pressed, however, it isn't phototoxic when steam distilled. Be aware of this before exposing yourself to UV or direct sunlight.

Lemongrass Oil

This type of essential oil has an earthy and lemon aroma to it. This oil is used for dealing with muscle aches, stress, oily skin, scabies, flatulence, excessive perspiration, acne, and athlete's foot.

This essential oil may have negative reactions when used with certain medication. If taking medication be sure to check any drug interactions before using. This oil should be avoided by children and should not be used on damaged skin.

Lime Oil

This type of essential oil has a tart and slightly citrus aroma to it. This oil is very affordable unlike some of the more expensive essential oils on this list. That makes it an ideal oil to add to your collection. This oil is mainly used for dealing with the flu, varicose veins, acne, colds, dull skin, and asthma.

This essential oil is phototoxic when cold pressed, however, it isn't phototoxic when steam distilled. Be aware of this before exposing yourself to UV or direct sunlight.

Marjoram Oil

This type of essential oil has a woody medicinal aroma to it. This oil is good for sprains, flatulence, excessive sex drive, muscle cramps, coughing, stress, hypertension, colic, bronchitis, ticks, and aching muscles.

This is a relatively safe and stable oil. No real precautions except not to misuse or abuse as are the case with all essential oils.

Melissa Oil

This type of essential oil has a fresh lemon aroma to it. This oil is great for fragrances, eczema, hypertension, depression, nausea, indigestion, asthma, insomnia, bronchitis, insect repellent, migraines, and menstrual cramping.

This essential oil may have a negative reaction when used with certain medication. If taking medication be sure to check any drug interactions before using. This oil should be avoided by children and should not be used on damaged skin.

Myrrh Oil

This essential oil has been around since Biblical times. This type of essential oil has a woody, warm, and earthy aroma to it. This oil is good for oral health and is used in rinses, mouthwash, and toothpaste. This oil also helps deal with chapped skin, bronchitis, toothache, ringworm, itching, hemorrhoids, halitosis, gum care, and athlete's foot.

This essential oil is fetotoxic and therefore should not be used by a woman who is pregnant or breastfeeding.

Myrtle Oil

This type of essential oil has a sweet slightly floral aroma to it. This oil is good for a sore throat, coughs, and asthma.

This essential oil may have a negative reaction when used with certain medication. If taking medication be sure to check any drug interactions before using. Research suggests this oil may be carcinogenic.

Neroli Oil

This type of essential oil has an intense floral and sweet aroma to it. This oil is ideal for dealing with depression, stretch marks, scars, stress, mature skin, insomnia, and shock.

This is a relatively safe and stable oil. No real precautions except not to misuse or abuse as are the case with all essential oils.

Niaouli Oil

This type of essential oil has a harsh, musty, earthy aroma to it. This oil is good for treating colds, coughs, bronchitis, whooping cough, sore throats, oily skin, acne, flu, and aches.

This oil should not be used around young children, especially near their faces as it can cause breathing issues and CNS.

Opoponax Oil

This type of essential oil has a deep woody aroma to it. This oil is ideal as an antispasmodic and antiseptic. This oil is known to help balance and mellow out emotions. It's used in a lot of incense and spiritual applications.

This essential oil is phototoxic. Be sure to avoid sunlight and other UV rays after applying topically. This oil is also a skin irritant and must be used with caution.

Orange Oil

This type of essential oil has a sweet orange aroma to it. This is a very popular and affordable essential oil. It is ideal for slow digestion, gums, flatulence, stress, constipation, colds, and dull skin. Orange oil is good for brightening one's mood and is also great for use in cleaning product recipes.

This is a relatively safe and stable oil. No real precautions except not to misuse or abuse as are the case with all essential oils.

Oregano Oil

This type of essential oil has a sharp and herb like aroma to it. This oil is great for both digestion and coughing.

This essential oil should be avoided by both children and by women who are pregnant or breastfeeding. This oil can cause skin irritation and mucous membrane irritation. This oil can also lead to blood clotting issues. Be very careful when using these oils. Do not use more than is called for in a recipe.

Palmarosa Oil

This type of essential oil has a fresh sweet floral aroma to it. This oil is perfect for hydrating the skin, aiding in digestion, and emotional contentment. Palmarosa oil has strong antiseptic and antibacterial properties. It's good at combating nervousness, fatigue, and stress related conditions.

This essential oil may have negative reactions when used with certain medication. If taking medication be sure to check any drug interactions before using.

Palo Santo Oil

This type of essential oil has a sweet woody yet slightly minty aroma to it. This oil is ideal for eliciting a sense of serenity and calm. It works great at fighting depression, emotional trauma, anxiety, coughs, colds, respiratory ailments, and even as an insect repellent.

This essential oil can cause skin irritation when applied topically. Be very careful when using these oils. Do not use more than is called for in a recipe.

Parsley Oil

This type of essential oil has a woody aroma to it. This oil is great for indigestion, arthritis, frigidity, and rheumatism.

This essential oil should be avoided by women who are pregnant or breastfeeding. This essential oil may have negative reactions when used with certain medication. If taking medication be sure to check any drug interactions before using.

Patchouli Oil

This type of essential oil has a rich earthy aroma to it. This oil is wonderful for skin care and is great in diffuser blends for romance. This is a personal favorite of mine and I use it all the time. This oil is ideal for stress, oily skin, eczema, mature skin, dermatitis, acne, chapped skin, athlete's foot, and as an insect repellent.

This essential oil may have a negative reaction when used with certain medication. If taking medication be sure to check any drug interactions before using. This oil may also inhibit blood clotting. Always be sure to use this oil carefully.

Peppermint Oil

This type of essential oil has a minty fresh aroma to it. This oil is known for having a cooling and calm effect. This oil is ideal for increasing mental alertness, increasing energy levels, aiding in digestion, reducing appetite, and elevating mood. This oil is also good for treating tension headaches, flatulence, vertigo, scabies, asthma, and colic. This oil is often considered to be an aphrodisiac.

This oil can cause skin irritation and mucous membrane irritation. This oil should not be used on children or people with certain medical heart conditions.

Petitgrain Oil

This type of essential oil has a fresh floral aroma to it. This oil is ideal for people dealing with stress, fatigue, oily skin, and acne. This oil is great for improving mood and providing a burst of energy.

This is a relatively safe and stable oil. No real precautions except not to misuse or abuse as are the case with all essential oils.

Ravensara Oil

This type of essential oil has a sweet and medicinal aroma to it. This oil is great for dealing with cold sores, influenza, joint pain, muscle pain, shingles, colds, and bronchitis.

Only use Ravensara oil that comes from the leaf. Do not use if it comes from the bark. This oil can cause skin irritation if not used properly.

Roman Chamomile Oil

This type of essential oil has a crisp, bright and fruity aroma to it. This oil is excellent for the sense of calm it can bring to those using it. This oil is ideal for dealing with insomnia, arthritis, stress, sprains, nausea, strains, cuts, boils, flatulence, earaches, colic, headaches, inflamed skin, rheumatism, sores, insect bites, abscesses, and allergies.

This is a relatively safe and stable oil. No real precautions except not to misuse or abuse as are the case with all essential oils.

Rose Geranium Oil

This type of essential oil has a floral aroma to it. This oil is ideal for dealing with menopause, dull skin, acne, lice, and oily skin.

This essential oil may have a negative reaction when used with certain medication. If taking medication be sure to check any drug interactions before using.

Rosemary Oil

This type of essential oil has a fresh, sweet, and medicinal aroma to it. This oil is great for our emotional well-being and can help to boost mood, stimulate the mind, and invigorate the soul. This oil is excellent for skin care and hair care. This oil is ideal for dealing with gout, exhaustion, poor circulation, dandruff, aching muscles, arthritis, rheumatism, and muscle cramps.

This essential oil is potentially neurotoxic and should be not be used on children. This oil can cause skin irritation if not used properly.

Rosewood Oil

This type of essential oil has a sweet, fruity, and woody aroma to it. Rosewood is a great aromatic oil. This oil is ideal for dealing with sensitive skin, stress, scars, flu, fever, acne, colds, and stretch marks.

This is a relatively safe and stable oil. No real precautions except not to misuse or abuse as are the case with all essential oils.

Sandalwood Oil

This type of essential oil has a rich, delicate, and sweet aroma to it. Sandalwood is great for instilling a sense of calm and inner peace. This oil is ideal for dealing with scars, oily skin, depression, bronchitis, laryngitis, stretch marks, dry skin, and stress.

This essential oil can cause skin irritation in rare instances. Be careful not to misuse or abuse the use of this essential oil.

Spearmint Oil

This type of essential oil has a minty and fruity aroma to it. This oil is great for easing headaches and tension. This oil is ideal for exhaustion, scabies, flatulence, asthma, vertigo, and fever.

This oil can cause skin irritation and mucous membrane irritation. Always be sure to use this oil carefully.

Spruce Oil

This type of essential oil has a sweet, earthy, and woody aroma to it. This oil is great for dealing with depression and coughing.

This is a relatively safe and stable oil. No real precautions except not to use the oil once it has gotten old and oxidized.

Tree Tea Oil

This type of essential oil has a medicinal and earthy aroma to it. Tree Tea is one of my favorite oils and I always keep it close by. This oil is great for cold sores, candida, warts, sores, insect bites, oily skin, colds, flu, whooping cough, migraines, itching, and sinusitis.

This essential oil can cause skin irritation in rare instances. Be careful not to misuse or abuse the use of this essential oil.

Thyme Oil

This type of essential oil has a fresh and medicinal aroma to it. This oil is ideal for dealing with MRSA, colds, arthritis, cuts, lice, poor circulation, oily skin, sore throat, laryngitis, dermatitis, and muscle aches.

This is a relatively safe and stable oil. No real precautions except not to misuse or abuse as are the case with all essential oils.

Vetiver Oil

This type of essential oil has a smokey, woody, and earthy aroma to it. This oil is great for spiritual and emotional applications. Vetiver oil is very strong and should always be diluted. This oil is ideal for dealing with stress, rheumatism, cuts, arthritis, depression, rheumatism, sores, oily skin, insomnia, and acne.

This essential oil can cause skin irritation in some instances. Be careful not to misuse or abuse the use of this essential oil.

Yarrow Oil

This type of essential oil has a sharp woody aroma to it. This oil is great for dealing with scars, indigestion, hair care, fever, varicose veins, insomnia, hypertension, hemorrhoids, wounds, and stretch marks.

This essential oil may have a negative reaction when used with certain medication. If taking medication be sure to check any drug interactions before using. This oil is also potentially neurotoxic and can cause skin irritation in some cases.

Ylang Ylang Oil

This type of essential oil has a sweet, fruity, and floral aroma to it. One of my personal favorites this oil is ideal for combating oily skin and acne, reducing stress, and as an aphrodisiac. This oil is good for dealing with hypertension, depression, anxiety, stress and palpitations.

This essential oil should be avoided by children. This oil can cause skin irritation and should not be used on damaged skin or hypersensitive skin.

Chapter Three: Essential Oil Safety & Hazardous Essential Oils

Essential Oil Safety

Essential oils can be harmful if not handled appropriately. These are highly concentrated liquids and are very powerful even in small doses. This power means when used correctly they can be extremely beneficial. Unfortunately if used in an improper manner they can have dangerous side effects. Implementing essential oils into your lifestyle doesn't need to be a stressful or worrisome situation, but it's important that you learn about using these oils safely and in an appropriate manner. By treating the use of essential oils with caution and respect, you'll be on your way to safely benefiting from all that these wonderful oils have to offer.

This section on safety is by no way a complete safety reference guide. Every oil has its own set of rules you'll want to abide by. Always be sure to research the oils your using before actually using them. If you're ever in doubt I suggest consulting a trained aromatherapy practitioner or your doctor. It's always best to err on the side of caution. The last thing you want to do is cause more harm than good. The whole point of using essential oils is to improve your life.

Essential oils shouldn't ever be used on your skin undiluted While an experienced user or trained professional may make exceptions to this rule on occasion, someone newer to essential oils should never make that attempt on their own. Many times you'll see people say that tea tree oil and lavender oil can be used undiluted. I suggest not trying this as a certain percentage of people will still suffer from a severe reaction to the undiluted oil. It's better to be safe and **NEVER** use any type of essential oil undiluted.

When you apply an essential oil for the first time on your skin, I suggest using a skin patch test on a tiny area of your skin to make sure you're not allergic or sensitive to the oil. Everyone is different. Certain oils will affect people in different ways. No one's body chemistry is exactly the same. It's always best to test before jumping in.

Essential oils aren't highly regulated. This means knowing exactly what is in each bottle is hard to know. This makes buying only high-quality essential oils from known and respected companies very important. Don't go with a company that has no reputation or a bad reputation. You need to have confidence that you're getting what you paid for when buying your essential oils. I go over a few of the places I use and trust in a later chapter.

Another thing to be aware of is that some types of essential oils are what is known as phototoxic. What is that you ask? Well, this means these oils can cause inflammation, redness, burning, and irritation when they get exposed to any UVA rays. You'll see in a few of the recipes I've included that I mention not to go directly into the sunlight once you've applied it topically. This is because they contain phototoxic oils which can lead to one of the side effects above. Always be sure to check the side effects of essential oils before using them. You also want to check if they have any harmful interactions when mixed with other specific oils or drugs.

There are many types of essential oils that need to be avoided by certain groups of people. For instance, children and pregnant women have certain oils they should not be using. Also, people suffering from certain health conditions like epilepsy and asthma will need to steer clear of certain essential oils. Don't forget to check an essential oils safety information before using it.

Many people underestimate the strength of essential oils. This is one of those things where less is definitely more. When using these oils you want to always use the least amount that will get the job you're trying to accomplish done. If a recipe calls for 2 drops, only use 2 drops. These oils are very concentrated and using more than what is called for can have unintended side effects or just be wasteful.

Don't get suckered in by people or businesses telling you to use as much of their products in one sitting as you'd like. Those people are trying to improve their bottom line. They are not thinking about your overall well-being. The faster you go through your oils the quicker you'll need to reorder more. Essential oils are not inexpensive. Be mindful of this when using them. Your wallet will thank you.

Do not use any of the hazardous oils I'll go over later in this chapter. These oils can be dangerous and if used, should only be done so by an experienced aromatherapy practitioner. Even then I suggest avoiding these oils. There's no need to put your health or well-being at risk.

Always keep children away from your essential oils. Keep your oils stored in a safe and secure location within your home. Many oils have a pleasant smell and unsuspecting children will think they are safe to ingest or use in a large amount, undiluted on their skin. Treat your essential oils like they were prescription medicine. They can be very dangerous in the hands of those not educated on how to use them.

When first starting out never take essential oils internally without consulting an expert or physician first. This may change once you've gained enough experience but it's not worth the risk when you don't fully grasp everything involved. People new to essential oils will often get the dosage or recipe wrong and end up harming themselves. Don't let this be you!

Don't forget that essential oils are very flammable. Always keep them away from open flames and other fire hazards. Be diligent with this. I've heard a few horror stories over the years. It's a simple precaution to take but one with steep consequences if ignored.

6 Factors Influencing The Safety of Essential Oils

Most of this I discussed above but here are 6 factors that can influence how safe the essential oils we use are. Knowing these will allow you to make smarter decisions when choosing the essential oils you want to incorporate into your daily life.

1. Quality

The less pure an essential oil the more likely you'll have an adverse response to it. Always try and use the purest essential oils you can find. The more authentic the better off you'll be.

2. Application Method

Essential oils can be used in a variety of ways. They can be applied topically, diffused, inhaled, and ingested. Each one of these methods has their own set of safety issues to contend with. Ingestion can be the most dangerous. Ingesting the wrong type or amount of oil can lead to coma and even death. When applying topically one must make sure that they are not sensitive or allergic to the oil in question. You'll also want to check the phototoxicity of an oil and whether it has any harmful interactions when mixed with other oils or medications. Topically applied oil can cause irritation and even burns when not used correctly. Diffusion and inhalation have the lowest risks associated with them. In more extreme cases you may begin to get headaches, lethargy, vertigo, and nausea when using them incorrectly.

3. Dosage

Always be sure to use the right amount of oil. Never use more than what is called for. Doing so will only increase the level of danger. Always dilute your oil when using topically. Blending oils and carrier oils can mitigate the negative effects they may have otherwise.

4. Chemical Composition

Essential oils rich in aldehydes and phenols may at times cause bad skin reactions. Essential oils that are rich in those kind of constituents should always be diluted prior to any application on the skin. Always be aware of the chemical composition of the oils you choose to use.

5. Skin Integrity

Damaged, inflamed, or diseased skin is more permeable to essential oils and can be much more sensitive to a dermal reaction. It's potentially very dangerous to put any undiluted essential oils on your damaged, inflamed, or diseased skin. Under that kind of circumstance, one's skin condition may become worse, and a larger amount of the oil will be absorbed than is normally. The rate of sensitization reactions will also rise on damaged, inflamed, and diseased skin.

6. Age & Health

Infants and younger children are much more sensitive to the potency of various essential oils than adults are. The same can be said for elderly users, pregnant women, and people suffering from certain medical conditions. Always know what types of oils are appropriate for the people using them. Just because it's safe for you doesn't mean that applies to everyone else.

Essential Oils That Are Phototoxic

Stay out of the sun or tanning beds after applying one of these essential oils to your skin for at least 24 hours. Otherwise, you could have an adverse reaction such as burning, irritation, and skin pigmentation changes.

Angelica Root

Bergamot

Cumin

Distilled or Expressed Grapefruit

Expressed Lemon

Expressed Lime

Orange Bitter

Rue

Essential Oils to Avoid During Pregnancy

Avoid using these essential oils at any time during your pregnancy. These can all have harmful side effects.

Aniseed

Basil

Birch

Camphor

Carrot Seed

Cassia

Cinnamon Bark

Clary Sage

Hyssop

Lemongrass

Mugwort

Parsley Seed or Leaf

Pennyroyal

Rosemary

Sage

Tansy

Tarragon

Thuja

Thyme

Vetiver

White Fir

Wintergreen

Wormwood

Essential Oils That Are Mucous Membrane Irritants

Do not use any of these essential oils in baths. These mucous membrane irritants can produce a drying and heating effect on the membranes of your nose, mouth, eyes, and reproductive organs.

Bay

Caraway

Cinnamon Bark or Leaf

Clove Bud or Leaf

Lemongrass

Peppermint

Thyme

Commonly Misused Essential Oils

Essential oils are dangerous if they get misused. Here are a few examples of essential oils that can cause serious health issues when used incorrectly.

Camphor Oil

This type of essential oil is often used as a moth repellent or as an ingredient in skin preparations. Even a tiny amount of camphor is extremely dangerous if swallowed. Seizures can begin almost immediately. Camphor poisoning can also occur when applied topically on children in higher doses than recommended on the label or if the child is covered in a bunch of extra clothing.

Eucalyptus Oil

This type of essential oil is used for the soothing effects it has when inhaled. For example, during a cold or a bad cough. If this oil is swallowed it can cause seizures.

Nutmeg Oil

This type of essential oil is used in food but, if abused or misused, it can cause vivid hallucinations and even lead to a coma.

Peppermint Oil

This type of essential oil is often used to relieve gastrointestinal discomfort. It's very important to choose the correct species of mint you'll be using as some types of these are poisonous. For example, pennyroyal oil is extremely poisonous to our livers.

<u>Sage Oil</u>

This type of essential oil is often used as a seasoning, scent, or remedy. Swallowing more than a tiny amount can cause seizures in children.

Hazardous Essential Oils

Here is a list of some of the hazardous essential oils you should avoid using altogether. These are different than the oils I described above. These oils should always be avoided. Not all people do this. You may come across some of these oils being used in recipes by other people. That doesn't mean it's safe for you to use. An experienced practitioner may be able to use some of these oils but even then it is risky. Someone just starting out should absolutely steer clear of these essential oils. There's plenty of safer options available. There's no need to risk your well being using any of the oils listed below. Please don't assume that an essential oil is safe because it isn't included down below. This is by no means a definitive list.

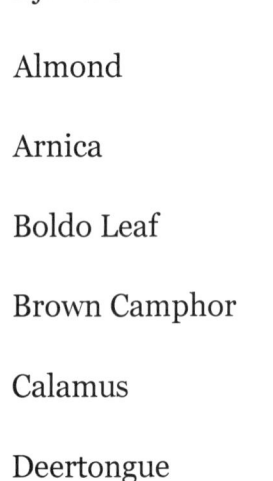

Ajowan

Almond

Arnica

Boldo Leaf

Brown Camphor

Calamus

Deertongue

Garlic

Horseradish

Jaborandi

Melilotus

Mugwort

Mustard

Onion

Pennyroyal

Rue

Sassafras

Spanish Broom

Sweet Birch

Thuja

Wintergreen

Wormseed

Wormwood

Yellow Camphor

Chapter Four: A Guide to Essential Oils Tools, Resources, Apps, & Books

Essential Oils Tools Guide

Getting started with essential oils can feel overwhelming at first. I often get asked what you types of items one should have when first starting out. In this section, I'm going to go over some of the main things I suggest picking up, along with some other items you can add along the way as you advance and get more comfortable. Feel free to pick and choose what you think will best suit you and your specific set of needs from the list I've provided. These are just some of the items I'm personally familiar with. If you have a preferred brand, by all means, get what makes the most sense to you. Everyone is different! My taste in essential oils will probably differ from yours. It's all about experimenting and finding the oils and tools that you get the most benefit from.

Accessories

2 oz Blue Glass Jars w/ Lids - Great colored jars w/ lids for your essential oils. I get mine off Amazon. Costs about $12.99

2 oz PET Plastic Jars w/ Lids - Excellent plastic jars. Have a variety of uses. I get mine off Amazon. Costs about $19.99.

2 oz Plastic Spray Bottles - Everyone should own a set of these cobalt blue plastic spray bottles. I get mine off Amazon. Costs about $12.95.

Amber Glass Bottles - I use these type of bottles all the time. I get mine off Amazon. Costs about $6.99.

Beeswax – I use Chefland Organic Beeswax. Costs about $6.25.

Blank Nasal Inhaler Tubes - Set of 24. Great for aromatherapy. I get mine off Amazon. Costs about $13.99.

Cotton Balls – I use Swisspers Organic Cotton Balls. Contains 80 balls. Costs about $5.65.

Deodorant Containers - Pack of 5 empty containers. I get mine off Amazon. Costs about $6.95.

Diffusers - There are a million options for diffusers. You can find these on some of the sites listed below or off Amazon.

Diffuser Jewelry - Lots of options to choose from. You can find these on some of the sites listed below or off Amazon.

Droppers - Pack of 12 glass droppers. I get mine off Amazon. Costs around $7.70.

Empty Capsules – I get 250 empty capsules at a time. I get mine off Amazon Costs around $8.75.

Epsom Salt – I go for the 5lb pound bag off Amazon. Costs around $14.99.

Funnel - Great item to have handy. I get mine off Amazon. Costs around $2.00.

Glass Beakers - Set of 3 Karter Scientific SF-214T2 Borosilicate Glass Beaker Set, 50/100/250 mL. Costs around $7.85.

Glass Mixing Bowls - Pyrex Prepware 3-Piece Glass Mixing Bowl Set. Costs around $12.95.

Mixing Glass Stir Rods - Good item to have around. I use rods that are 200mm 8-inch. Comes in a pack of 12. I get mine off Amazon. Costs around $9.25.

Labels - I use Mudder Fancy Kraft Paper Essential Oil Bottle Stickers Labels, 6 Sheets. Costs around $8.99.

Lip Balm Tubes - Set of 50 generic empty tubes. I get mine off Amazon. Costs around $9.00.

Notebook - Any notebook will do but I use a Moleskine Classic Notebook. Costs around $15.50.

Paper Towels - Any type will do. I prefer using these Bounty paper towels. Costs around $20.00.

Shea Butter - I love this stuff. I use Viva Naturals Organic Shea Butter. Costs around $12.95.

Silicone Molds - There are a large variety of molds available but I mainly use Milliard 5.5cm. Steel Bath Bomb Molds. Costs around $6.99.

Storage Box - A must have for anyone who uses essential oils. I use a SOLIGT 25 Slot Wooden Essential Oil Box. Costs around $14.95.

Travel Case - I love having a travel case for when I go away. Comes in handy. I got mine off Amazon. Costs around $34.95.

Wool Dryer Balls - A great item to have in your arsenal. I use Smart Sheep 6-Pack, XL Premium Reusable Natural Wool Dryer Balls. Costs around $18.95.

Oils

There's a ton of different essential oils out there. In this section, I'm going to provide some of the main carrier oils I use and some of the most popular essential oils. I suggest always doing your own research and going with a brand that works best for you. These are just the one's that I've used and that I'm familiar with. Remember these are just some to get started with. There's plenty of other oils to experiment with once you've gotten up and running.

Carrier Oils

Coconut Oil – I use Nature's Oil 76 Degree Coconut Oil. Leaves an oily feeling on the top layer of skin. Solid white color at room temperature. Has a coconut aroma to it. Has a long nearly indefinite shelf life. Costs around $4.00.

Fractionated Coconut Oil – I use Nature's Oil Fractionated Coconut Oil. Has a non-greasy consistency. Liquid at room temperature. Has no aroma to it. Absorbs nicely leaving skin feeling silky. Has a long nearly indefinite shelf-life. Costs around $7.00.

Grapeseed Oil – I use Nature's Oil Grapeseed Oil. Has a nice thin and light consistency. Nearly odorless. Good for essential oil massages. Has a shorter shelf life of 6 to 12 months. Costs around $5.50.

Jojoba Oil – I use Nature's Oil Golden Jojoba Oil. Has a medium consistency. Has a nutty aroma to it. Good for moisturizing your hair and skin. Has a long nearly indefinite shelf life. Costs around $7.25.

Olive Oil – I use Nature's Oil Extra-Virgin Olive Oil. Has a thick oily consistency. Comes with a powerful aroma. Good for both culinary and topical essential oil applications. Has a shorter shelf life of 1 to 2 years. Costs around $7.25.

Sweet Almond Oil – I use Nature's Oil Sweet Almond Oil. Has a medium consistency. Has a nutty, slightly sweet aroma to it. Absorbs quickly and moisturizes well. Not ideal for people with allergies to nuts. Has around a 12-month shelf life. Costs around $5.75.

Essential Oils

Bergamot Oil - Great for reducing anxiety. Works wonders on the skin. I use DoTERRA Bergamot Oil. Costs around $37.00.

Cinnamon Bark Oil - Great aromatic oil. I enjoy this one quite a bit. I use Young Living Cinnamon Bark Oil. Costs around $32.00.

Clary Sage Oil - Good for sleep and great for your hair and scalp. I use DoTERRA Clary Sage Oil. Costs around $49.00.

Eucalyptus Oil - Promotes a clear mind and feelings of relaxation. I use DoTERRA Eucalyptus Oil. Costs around $19.00.

Frankincense Oil – This is a powerful oil that's great for both emotional support and skincare. I use Young Living Frankincense Oil. Costs around $97.00.

Grapefruit Oil - Helps with metabolism and is wonderful mood uplifter. I use DoTERRA Grapefruit Oil. Costs around $22.00.

Lavender Oil – Great beginner oil. Promotes healthy skin, relaxation, and stress relief. I use Young Living Lavender Oil. Costs around $32.00.

Lemon Oil – Lemon is an awesome deodorizer that can cut grease and be used to help keep your home and clothes feeling fresh and clean. I use Young Living Lemon Oil. Costs around $15.00.

Melaleuca Oil – Also known as Tea Tree Oil. This oil is a wonderful skin cleanser and helps to promote healthier immune function. I use DoTERRA Melaleuca Oil. Costs around $26.00.

Patchouli Oil - Helps to reduce wrinkles, skin imperfections, and blemishes. Also a good mood stabilizer. I use DoTERRA Patchouli Oil. Costs around $40.00.

Peppermint Oil – Great for reducing tension and aiding with digestive issues. I use Young Living Peppermint Oil. Costs around $29.00.

Pine Oil - Very refreshing. I love the smell of pine so this is a personal favorite. I use Young Living Pine Oil. Costs around $20.00.

Vetiver Oil - Promotes a restful sleep and helps to keep one calmer and more grounded. I use DoTERRA Vetiver Oil. Costs around $46.00.

Wild Orange Oil - Excellent cleanser and provides needed antioxidants. Good for improving mood. I use DoTERRA Wild Orange Oil. Costs around $14.00.

Ylang Ylang Oil - Great for both the skin and hair. Uplifts mood while still keeping one calm. I use DoTERRA Ylang Ylang Oil. Costs around $47.00.

Essential Oils Resource Guide

In this section, I will go over my favorites sites and resources related to essential oils. There's a wealth of information on the subject. If you have a question, I'd be surprised if you couldn't find it using one of these resources.

Aroma Web - Probably my favorite site to learn about essential oils and find recipes.

http://www.aromaweb.com/

Bulk Apothecary - Great site. Have purchased from here many times in the past.

http://www.bulkapothecary.com/

DoTERRA - One of my favorite sites to purchase essential oils. Love the quality and selection of what they offer.

http://doterra.com/US/en

Essential Oils Haven - Article comparing some of the top essential oil brands. Nice breakdown to give you an idea of how the top essential oils companies compare to one another.

http://www.essentialoilhaven.com/best-essential-oil-brands/

Life Science - Has a lot of helpful products and books dealing with essential oils. I've gotten a few of my diffusers from this site in the past.

http://www.discoverlsp.com/

Mountain Rose Herbs - A good site offering a variety of essential oils and accessories for sale.

http://www.mountainroseherbs.com/catalog/aromatherapy/essential-oils

NAHA - Stands for the National Association for Holistic Aromatherapy. Wonderful organization with links to all types of articles, resources, seminars, career opportunities, and books on essential oils and aromatherapy. An excellent resource site and one I suggest everyone take a look at.

http://naha.org/

Young Living - A wonderful site where I purchase many of my essential oils from. Lots of information, articles, and products to choose from.

https://www.youngliving.com/en_US

Essential Oils App Guide

In this section, I'm going to discuss my favorite apps related to essential oils These are apps that I've tried out myself at one point. I'm sure there are others I may have missed but this guide will give you a good idea of the different apps available to you. I suggest trying a few and sticking with those that best suit your needs.

Ref Guide For Essential Oils - Costs $6.99. Available on both iOS and Android. One of my favorites. Presents an in-depth look at essential oils.

Best Essential Oils & Aromatherapy Guide Pro - Free app available on the iOS. Offers a ton of information on essential oils. Excellent reference app.

Essential Oils & More - Free app available on the Android. Offers a comprehensive guide to the world of essential oils.

Modern Essentials - Costs $6.99. Available on both iOS and Android. Another wonderful app. Found it to be well laid out and easy to navigate.

Essential Oils Book Guide

Here are a few of my favorite books on essential oils. I've read a lot on this subject over the years and these are a few of the books that made an impression. I hope they do the same for you.

1. **The Complete Book of Essential Oils and Aromatherapy** by Valerie Ann Worwood

2. **Essential Oils Natural Remedies: The Complete A-Z Reference of Essential Oils for Health and Healing** by Althea Press

3. **The Complete Aromatherapy and Essential Oils Handbook for Everyday Wellness** by Nerys Purchon & Lora Cantele

4. **Essential Oil Safety: A Guide for Health Care Professionals** by Robert Tisserand & Rodney Young

5. **Gentle Babies Essential Oils and Natural Remedies for Pregnancy, Childbirth, Infants and Young Children** by Debra Raybern

6. **The Encyclopedia of Essential Oils** by Julia Lawless

7. **Reference Guide for Essential Oils** by Connie & Alan Higley

Chapter Five: Essential Oils FAQ / Common Terms & Meanings

Essential Oils Frequently Asked Questions (FAQ)

In this section, I will go over some of the common questions I come across the most when talking about essential oils. I hope you're able to find the answer to whatever remaining questions you have. If I missed something you should be able to find it on one of the sites or books I recommended in the previous chapter.

1. What Things Should I Look For When It Comes To Essential Oils?

When using your essential oils, one should use the highest quality oils you can reasonably afford.

I recommend looking for companies that grow the plants they use in their oils without using any pesticides. A certified organic company is always my preference. You can usually find out if the company you're thinking of using meets those standards by visiting their website or contacting them directly.

While many companies make essential oils that are actually pure enough to be ingested internally, many essential oils made are diluted with a carrier oil or were derived from plants grown with pesticides. Those oils you wouldn't want to ingest internally.

You should seek out oils that have been tested for their purity before being sold. The purer the oil the better. I prefer oils without any additives in them, like carrier oils.

2. How Do I Go About Using Essential Oils?

Essential oils can be used in a variety of different ways. Here are the main ones:

Internally - A select amount of higher quality essential oils are safe for internal use.

Topically – Many essential oils are meant to be applied directly on your skin, diluting them with a carrier oil.

Aromatically – Diffusing your essential oils in the air around you is a wonderful way to get all the benefits of the essential oils. I have diffusers in each room of my home so I can always use my oils whenever the need arises.

3. Can I Ingest Essential Oils?

As I mentioned in the last two questions, you can ingest some essential oils, however, in general, I would suggest avoiding that. Always be sure to vet a company that suggests taking their oils internally and be sure to follow the instructions carefully. If you have any doubts, I'd suggest not taking them or contact the company directly for more information.

If your essential oils are safe to consume you can try taking them using a few different methods:

Capsule – Many companies sell empty capsules online or in your neighborhood health food store. Capsules are an excellent way of taking essential oils that would normally burn your mouth if you take them in water or undiluted.

Underneath Your Tongue – Many types of essential oils, like your digestive essential oil blends, are best taken under your tongue. Simply start with a single drop, see how you're feeling after a couple of minutes and take another drop if you need it. Relief should happen pretty quickly.

In Your Water – Many types of essential oils, like wild orange, lemon, and peppermint, are perfect in water. The typical dilution is approximately 1 drop per 4 ounces of water.

4. How Often Can I Use Essential Oils?

This is a question I often hear a lot of different answers to. Personally, I recommend using essential oils on a needed basis. By doing this you're preventing your body from becoming too accustomed to whatever ailment you're trying to remedy. For essential oils that you need to use on regular basis, like those for sleep, I recommend alternating the types of calming oils you use.

5. What Is A Carrier Oil?

This is an oil that you use as a base in order to dilute other essential oils before you apply them to your skin. Diluting essential oils is always a good idea when you're using them.

6. How Are Essential Oils Used With Children?

There are certain essential oils that are toxic to kids if taken in a large enough dose. For example, large doses of wintergreen or small doses taken internally of melaleuca. Therefore it's important that you treat your essential oils like they were medication and store them out of the reach of your kids. You also should teach them about how to properly use essential oils so if they do get into them they know how to safely use them.

Whenever I use essential oils on the children I'm always sure to dilute them in either a tub of bathwater or carrier oil. I also try and apply the oils to the bottoms of their feet. The reason behind this is because while the oil still enters the bloodstream quickly, the tougher skin on the bottom of feet isn't prone to getting irritated like most other parts of the body are.

Another tip is to watch over them while they learn to apply the oils themselves. I dilute the oil for them first while they watch but I like to let them apply it so that they can learn to do it for themselves when they are older.

7. Which Types Of Essential Oils Are Safe For Pregnant Women?

Using essential oils during pregnancy requires a little more caution. For instance, be very careful of what you use during the first few weeks of your pregnancy as this is a rapid time of development for the baby. I've included some oils to avoid during pregnancy, but you should monitor yourself and the amount of oil you're using even if they aren't on this list.

Always dilute your oils while pregnant. Do not apply an oil directly to your skin before doing so. I suggest stick with aromatherapy whenever possible. Diffusing your oils aromatically is a much safer way to use your essential oils while pregnant. Most issues pregnant women have with essential oils during pregnancy arise from internal and topical use.

Essential Oils To Avoid During Pregnancy:

Aniseed

Basil

Birch

Camphor

Cassia

Cinnamon Bark

Clary Sage

Hyssop

Lemongrass

Mugwort

Parsley Seed or Leaf

Pennyroyal

Rosemary

Sage

Tansy

Tarragon

Thuja

Thyme

Vetiver

White Fir

Wintergreen

Wormwood

8. Are Essential Oils Allowed While Still Breastfeeding?

The answer to this is yes. Just like in pregnancy this can be doing using some precautions. I've included a list of essential oils that are safe for you to use when breastfeeding.

Essential Oils Safe To Use When Breastfeeding:

Lemon

Ylang Ylang

Clary Sage

Bergamot

Geranium

Lavender

Patchouli

Grapefruit

Wild Orange

Sandalwood

Roman Chamomile

Peppermint (Only Sparingly)

9. What Types Of Precautions Do I Need To Take When Using Essential Oils?

Even though essential oils are natural, they tend to be extremely potent. I always advise using precaution when using them. Here are a few things I suggest doing when dealing with essential oils.

1. Keep them away from your eyes.

2. Only use higher quality oils whenever possible. The better the quality the purer they tend to be.

3. Always test the oils on your skin before using topically. You want to make sure you don't have a negative reaction before applying more liberally.

4. If you do have a negative reaction stop using that particular oil.

5. If you are ever in doubt about the strength of the oil be sure to dilute it.

6. See how your body reacts. If something feels wrong, immediately stop using that essential oil.

10. What Amount Of Essential Oil Should I Be Using?

A tiny amount can go a long way. Work your way up from one drop unless using a specific recipe that recommends you do otherwise.

11. How Can You Determine The Quality Of An Essential Oil?

There are a ton of variables that will come into play when determining the quality of an essential oil. Here are some of the things that can affect the quality.

1. Altitude and climate where it was originally grown.

2. The amount of rainfall.

3. The quality of the soil.

4. How it got harvested.

5. Time passed between being harvested and distilled.

6. How it got stored before being distilled.

7. The reputation of the company selling the oil. Certain companies are known for producing high-grade essential oils, while other less reputable companies may try blending pure essential oils with lower quality oils. Some of these less than reputable companies may also try and add synthetic constituents to their oil in an attempt to "improve" the low quality.

12. What Types Of Items Are Needed To Properly Use Essential Oils?

I went over all the types of tools I use in the last chapter. However, here are a few you may find helpful having right from the beginning.

Bottles

Droppers

Cotton Balls

Diffusers

Carrier Oil

Reference Guide

13. How Long Will Essential Oils Last?

I often get asked if essential oils will last "forever". Unfortunately, the answer to that is no. Essential oils tend to be volatile, the more you open the bottle they are stored in the faster all the constituents in your oil will begin to evaporate.

Like many items, the shelf life of your essential oils will depend on the type of oil and the manner in which they are stored. Here are a few tips to help improve the shelf life of your essential oils.

1. Close the bottle lids tightly after every use.

2. Keep them away from light. I have a storage cabinet I hold most of my oils in.

3. Keep them cool. I have many friends who refrigerate their oils in mini fridges. I wouldn't suggest mixing them in with where you keep anything you'll be ingesting.

Many citrus oils have a shelf life of between 1 and 3 years, while more woodsy oils can last for closer to a decade. If your oil ever begins to thicken, smell differently or appear cloudy it's time to discard it. Better to be safe than sorry.

Essential Oils Common Terms & Meanings

Here is a list of some essential oils terms & meanings you may run across at certain points. You don't need to memorize these or remember them all by heart but it would be a good idea to at least familiarize yourself with this list. It also acts a nice reference point if you don't remember the meaning of something.

Anti-Fungal - Claims the ability to prevent and treat fungal infections and fungal growth. Always check any facts being claimed against any types of credible studies you can find. Just because something claims to be anti-fungal doesn't always means it's true.

Anti-Inflammatory - Helps to reduce the amount of inflammation.

Antineuralgic - Prevents and inhibits sharp pains from occurring along the nerves.

Antiphlogistic - Helps to reduce inflammation and can also sometimes include fever relief.

Antiseptic - This indicates that the ingredient is pure and clean. That it helps to prevent the growth of microbial or other disease-inducing agents.

Antispasmodic - Helps to relieve spasms that may occur in our involuntary muscles. These include our heart and intestines.

Aperitif - This is a type of essential oil that helps work to stimulate a person's appetite.

Aphrodisiac - This is something that helps to titillate or stimulate sexual desire, excitement, and attraction.

Aromatherapy - This is a popular branch of holistic medicine that uses oils and plant material in an attempt to alter our mental prowess, mood, physical, and psychological well-being. This is considered an alternative medicine that has many studies showing it can have many powerful applications.

Astringent - A type of solution that can cause contractions in the tissues of your body. It's nearly universally used in tandem with the skin in health and wellness applications.

Bactericidal - A general term that included a bunch of agents that kill off bacteria. These include antiseptics, antibiotics, and disinfectants.

Cytophylactic - These are believed to protect our cells and fight infections. They increase leucocytes, which stimulant cellular repair and regeneration.

Depurative - A term that means that something has detoxifying and purifying properties. It helps cleanse away toxins and wastes from the system.

Disinfectant - A solution that has anti-microbial agents or properties.

Diuretic - Cause the boy to increase the passage and production of urine.

Emmenagogue - A term that refers to any type of substance that helps increase or stimulate menstrual flow. It can also indicate an increase in the blood flow to the uterus or pelvis.

Emollient - Anything that works to soothe or soften the skin.

Essential Oil - Refers to any number of different natural oils, which are normally obtained through the distillation process of a plant or other botanical. What gives these oils their properties is that they contain chemicals and volatile aroma compounds.

Expectorant - These work to promote the secretion of our mucus from our air passages. An expectorant encourages us to cough productively, in order to clear out our respiratory system and lungs.

Febrifuge - This is a term that means fever reducer.

Haemostatic - This is something that works to either stop or slows down the bleeding.

Hepatic - This term refers to any issues that relate to our liver.

Hypotensive - This term refers to something that lowers our blood pressure.

Lymphatic - This term refers to anything that has to do with our lymph. Lymph is a colorless fluid that contains our white blood cells and bathes all our tissues. It helps to drain from the lymphatic system into our bloodstream.

Nervine - This term refers to something that works to soothe or calm the nerves.

Neurotoxic - This term occurs when exposure to artificial or natural toxic substances, which are known as neurotoxins, alters the normal activity of your nervous system in a way that causes damage to our nervous tissue.

Phototoxicity - This term refers to a skin irritation that is chemically induced, requiring light, that does not involve our immune system. It is a type of photosensitivity. Our skin's response resembles that of an exaggerated sunburn.

Sedative - This term refers to an agent that works to induce sleep or promote a feeling of calm.

Stimulant - The opposite of a sedative. These raise your nervous and physical activity. For example, caffeine is a stimulant.

Stomachic - This is something that works to assist in digestion and promote appetite

Sudorific - This refers to something that is related to or helps causes you to sweat.

Tonic - This term refers to something that gives you a feeling of well-being or vigor.

Vermifuge - This term refers to something that works to help get rid of any parasitic worms in one's system.

Vulnerary - This term describes something used to help heal wounds.

Chapter Six: 50+ Quick Essential Oils Tips & Tricks

50+ Quick Essential Oils Tips & Tricks

In this section. I'll be going over a 50+ tips and tricks I've come across over my years using essential oils. Some of these you may already know but I find a good deal of them are new to most people. I hope they are able to help you the same way they've helped me.

1. To maximize the long-term effectiveness of essential oils take some short breaks from using them. For example, I like to take a day or two off from using them each week. Some people prefer to use them for a few weeks and then take off an entire week. Choose whatever way works best for you.

2. Never get essential oils into your eyes. If you do seek immediate help. Also avoid getting oils into your nose or ears.

3. Keep essential oils clear of dampness, light, heat, and all electromagnetic frequencies (microwaves, TV's).

4. If you don't like the smell of a particular essential oil do not use it for any emotional benefits. It won't have the intended effect.

5. It only takes an essential oil 1 second via inhalation or 3 seconds via skin application to reach your limbic system and start to kick in.

6. Lavender oil is good reducing the itching associated with bug bites and lessening the severity of migraines.

7. Myrrh, frankincense, and cinnamon are all thought to be strong anti-tumor and anti-cancer essential oils.

8. Avoid any tanning beds or strong sunlight after applying your essential oils. Especially when dealing with phototoxic oils.

9. Essential oils can help to renew our dying cells. That's why so many people use them for skin care.

10. Lemon, thyme, and clove essential oils are great natural disinfectants. In fact, they were often used in hospitals as disinfectants before the beginning of World War I.

11. Bergamot and clary sage oils help people withdrawing from alcohol, eating, or smoking addictions.

12. All types of essential oils are natural antioxidants.

13. Cinnamon oil has been known to help a home sell faster. If you're looking to list your property, try putting out some diffusers with cinnamon oil before holding your open houses.

14. You can make great heating pads out of rice and a large sock. Just add the rice to the sock and sew it shut. Scent with your essential oil and microwave to heat up when you have aches and pains.

15. Making your own essential oils all purpose cleaner is a wonderful way to incorporate more oils into your daily life. Just combine 2 parts water, 1 part vinegar, and 5 drops of your preferred essential oil in a glass spray bottle. Not only does it work great but it's cheap.

16. Using Aloe Vera will help to deepen the penetration of the essential oils into your joints, tissues, and muscles.

17. Add a few drops of essential oils to a new roll of toilet paper in order to keep your bathroom smelling nice.

18. Adding oils to wood dryer balls is a wonderful way to help fluff and separate laundry naturally. They break up static and keep the laundry smelling fresh. Great alternative to dryer sheets.

19. Whenever you change the air filters used in your HVAC, add in a few drops of your essential oils to help filter and freshen up the air as it is circulated through your house.

20. Frankincense oil can decrease an allergic reaction within mere seconds.

21. A great way to use essential oils is to wear your oils on jewelry. Diffuser necklaces and bracelets can easily be made at home or purchased from retailers. They normally last a full day before needing more oil added.

22. Keep your garbage can smelling fresh by dropping a cotton ball dabbed in essential oil to the bottom of your can in order to minimize odors.

23. Peppermint oil has been known to help people adapt easier to new ideas.

24. Perfume oils are not the same as essential oils. Many people get this confused. Perfume oils don't have any of the therapeutic benefits that essential oils offer.

25. Learn how to compare oils with the same names. Some plants have common names like lavender, anise, and eucalyptus. You need to always check the Latin botanical names to tell them apart. For example, two essential oils may be listed as lavender oil but they come from different plants. Since they come from different plants the aroma and properties of each oil may differ. The same can be said of the cost. Some will be more expensive because they are made from plants that are rare and hard to find.

26. Always store your oils in a cool, dark place away from the light. I keep multiple storage boxes so I can easily move my oils around as necessary.

27. Add a couple drops of essential oil to your hair rinse (approximately 5 to 7 drops in 1 cup of water). Massage it in thoroughly.

28. Add a couple of drops to your baking soda or cornstarch, mix and allow to set for a couple of days, then sprinkle it over your carpets. Allow to set for approximately an hour and then vacuum.

29. Always purchase your oils from a reputable company. I personally have used the Global Aromatherapy Business Directory in the past to find products and have been pleased with the results. Don't purchase oils from vendors you don't know. I often see people buy oils at craft shows and local fairs with no knowledge of the quality of the oil being purchased.

30. Fill your spray bottle with some water and add in a few drops of oil to use as a makeshift air freshener.

31. Add between 3 to 5 drops of your essential oil directly to your rinse water when washing your clothes.

32. Avoid purchasing essential oils that have rubber glass dropper tops. The reason for this is that essential oils are extremely concentrated and will turn the rubber into a gum-like substance which will ruin the essential oil.

33. You can add a few drops of essential oil to your old and worn out Potpourri in order to give it new life.

34. Add a single drop of lavender oil to the inside of your mascara tube to make it last longer and help promote thicker and longer lashes.

35. Put a few drops of your preferred essential oil onto your cotton ball and put it in a vacuum cleaner bag.

36. Place a drop or two of your essential oil into the melted hot wax of a candle that is burning. Does a great job of diffusing the oil.

37. All types of citrus essential oils will make your skin photosensitive.

38. Wax warmers are a cheap way to distribute your essential oils. Just fill your bowl with coconut oil and add a couple drops of your favorite oils. Once the warmer gets hot the oils will scent the air nicely.

39. Place a few drops of your lavender oil on a pillow in order to induce some sweet dreams.

40. Place a dab of your essential oil on a few cotton balls and place them all around your house in out of the way spots like drawers and closets.

41. You can place essential oils on light bulbs, scent rings, and radiators. Just be sure to avoid any electrical outlets or sockets.

42. Add 2 to 3 drops of your essential oil onto a dried log. Allow the oil to soak in and then place the log on the fire to diffuse.

43. You can diffuse essential oils in your tissue box in order to create scented tissues to help with your stuffy nose issues. Just open your box, add a few drops onto the tissues and close it back up.

44. Tea tree oils and lavender oils can be applied to your scrapes, cuts, or scratches for healing properties and pain relief.

45. Want a way to make a quick air freshener? Wood is porous so take some wooden clothes pins and place a few drops of essential oils on them. Then simply clip them anywhere you want to freshen up the air. Perfect for car air vents. You can also place your oil on wooden jewelry and wear your oils that way. If you don't have wood you can also use leather.

46. Put a couple of drops of your essential oil either directly into your shoes or try dabbing some onto a cotton ball and put one cotton ball in each of your shoes.

47. Create your own personalized perfume by adding between 10 to 25 drops of your preferred essential oil to 1 ounce of vodka or perfume alcohol.

48. Always pay attention to any warnings or safety precautions when dealing with essential oils. This is extremely important when dealing with children and woman who are pregnant.

49. Only cook with essential oils that are allowed to be ingested internally. Be sure to do your research.

50. Essential oils can have viscosity levels that differ from one another. When baking, don't drop your oil directly into your mix. Drop the amount called for on a spoon first and make sure you have the proper amount before adding. Essential oils are concentrated and powerful. You don't want to add more than what is called for.

51. You can create your own personalized bath salts using Epsom salts and your leftover bottles of essential oils. The salts will absorb the trace amounts of the essential oils left in your bottles. You can feel free to mix and match your scents. To use, add 2 to 4 tablespoons of your salts to any bath.

52. When applying oils for aromatic effects I suggest applying the oils to the skin close to your nose. You can also add it to the back of your neck, temples, the nose itself, wrists, or on a piece of jewelry.

53. Essential oils are flammable. Be careful to avoid any open flames, sparks, or electricity to avoid fire hazards.

54. Work with your essential oils in an area where you have a good source of ventilation. Overuse of your essential oils can lead to headaches or even dizziness so always be sure to take a break outdoors and work near an open window whenever possible.

55. To avoid any side effects or drug induced interactions be sure to consult your doctor before experimenting with essential oils. This is especially true if you're on medications as certain oils can heighten their effects.

Chapter Seven: 350+ Essential Oils Recipes

Essential Oils Recipes For Good Smelling Blends

Diffusing your essential oils will not only make your home smell nicer, it can also provide other health benefits. I always prefer to use cold-air diffusers. I prefer them because anything that heats your oils can do damage to some of their more beneficial properties. I suggest never using candle warmers or other items that can heat the essential oils excessively. Sticking with a cold air diffuser is the best way to ensure you benefit from all the positive effects of your essential oils.

In this section, I'll be going over essential oil recipes that are pleasant to smell. I've tried all of these at some point or another and have enjoyed them. Hopefully, you'll find a few that you enjoy as well.

Be aware the blends in this section are meant to be used in your cold-air diffuser. These types of diffusers will normally require a tiny amount of water to be added, along with any oils. Check your diffuser's directions to find out exact amounts necessary.

1. Citrus Forest Diffuser Recipe

2 Drops of Lemon Oil

2 Drops of Lime Oil

1 Drop of White Fir Oil

1 Drop of Bergamot Oil

1 Drop of Orange Oil

Directions:

Add these oils to your diffuser and enjoy.

2. Woodsy Feeling Diffuser Recipe

4 Drops of Frankincense Oil

3 Drops of White Fir Oil

2 Drops of Cedarwood Oil

Directions:

Add these oils to your diffuser and enjoy.

3. Clean & Fresh Diffuser Recipe

2 Drops of Rosemary Oil

2 Drops of Lemon Oil

2 Drops of Lavender Oil

Directions:

Add these oils to your diffuser and enjoy.

4. Citrus Bomb Diffuser Recipe

2 Drops of Wild Orange Oil

1 Drop of Lemon Oil

1 Drop of Grapefruit Oil

1 Drop of Lime Oil

Directions:

Add these oils to your diffuser and enjoy.

5. Spring & Summer Diffuser Recipe

2 Drops of Peppermint Oil

2 Drops of Lemon Oil

2 Drops of Lavender Oil

Directions:

Add these oils to your diffuser and enjoy.

6. The Candy Shop Diffuser Recipe

4 Drops of Wintergreen Oil

4 Drops of Wild Orange Oil

Directions:

Add these oils to your diffuser and enjoy.

7. Garden Flower Diffuser Recipe

2 Drops of Roman Chamomile Oil

2 Drops of Lavender Oil

1 Drop of Geranium Oil

Directions:

Add these oils to your diffuser and enjoy.

8. Christmas Magic Diffuser Recipe

4 Drops of Cinnamon Oil

4 Drops of Patchouli Oil

3 Drops of Orange Oil

2 Drops of Clove Oil

1 Drop of Ylang Ylang Oil

Directions:

Add these oils to your diffuser and enjoy.

9. Spicy Night Diffuser Recipe

4 Drops of Wild Orange Oil

3 Drops of Cinnamon Oil

2 Drops of Clove Oil

Directions:

Add these oils to your diffuser and enjoy.

10. Rugged Man Diffuser Recipe

2 Drops of Wintergreen Oil

2 Drops of Cypress Oil

2 Drops of White Fir Oil

Directions:

Add these oils to your diffuser and enjoy.

11. Chai Spice Diffuser Recipe

3 Drops of Cardamom Oil

2 Drops of Clove Oil

2 Drops of Cassia Oil

1 Drop of Ginger Oil

Directions:

Add these oils to your diffuser and enjoy.

12. Out In The Woods Diffuser Recipe

3 Drops of Frankincense Oil

2 Drops of White Fir Oil

1 Drop of Cedarwood Oil

Directions:

Add these oils to your diffuser and enjoy.

13. Citrus & Spice Diffuser Recipe

3 Drops of Wild Orange Oil

2 Drops of Cinnamon Bark Oil

1 Drop of Clove Oil

Directions:

Add these oils to your diffuser and enjoy.

14. Candy Dream Diffuser Recipe.

2 Drops of Wintergreen Oil

2 Drops of Wild Orange Oil

Directions:

Add these oils to your diffuser and enjoy.

15. Holiday Happiness Diffuser Recipe

2 Drops of Wild Orange Oil

2 Drops of White Fir Oil

1 Drop of Wintergreen Oil

Directions:

Add these oils to your diffuser and enjoy.

16. Autumn Breeze Diffuser Recipe

The feeling of fall weather.

8 Drops of Orange Oil

6 Drops of Sage Oil

6 Drops of Lime Oil

Directions:

Add these oils to your diffuser and enjoy.

17. Candy Cane Diffuser Recipe

3 Drops of Peppermint Oil

2 Drops of Vanilla Oil

Directions:

Add these oils to your diffuser and enjoy.

18. Spice & Cinnamon Diffuser Recipe

5 Drops of Vanilla Oil

1 Drop of Orange Oil

1 Drop of Nutmeg Oil

1 Drop of Clove Oil

1 Drop of Cinnamon Bark Oil

Directions:

Add these oils to your diffuser and enjoy.

19. Cinnamon, Spice & All That's Nice Diffuser Recipe

24 Drops of Cinnamon Cassia Oil

10 Drops of Ginger Oil

5 Drops of Orange Oil

4 Drops of Nutmeg Oil

Directions:

Add these oils to your diffuser and enjoy.

20. Fall Seasonal Blend Diffuser Recipe

4 Drops of Wild Orange Oil

3 Drops of Cinnamon Oil

3 Drops of Ginger Oil

Directions:

Add these oils to your diffuser and enjoy.

21. Summertime Seasonal Blend Diffuser Recipe

3 Drops of Lavender Oil

3 Drops of Grapefruit Oil

2 Drops of Spearmint Oil

2 Drops of Lemon Oil

Directions:

Add these oils to your diffuser and enjoy.

22. Spring Seasonal Blend Diffuser Recipe

3 Drops of Roman Chamomile Oil

3 Drops of Lavender Oil

2 Drops of Geranium Oil

Directions:

Add these oils to your diffuser and enjoy.

23. Winter Seasonal Blend Diffuser Recipe

3 Drops of Wild Orange Oil

3 Drops of White Fir Oil

2 Drops of Wintergreen Oil

Directions:

Add these oils to your diffuser and enjoy.

24. Man Cave Blend Diffuser Recipe

2 Drops of Wintergreen Oil

2 Drops of Cypress Oil

2 Drops of White Fir Oil

Directions:

Add these oils to your diffuser and enjoy.

25. Fresh Fallen Snow Diffuser Recipe

6 Drops of Grapefruit Oil

2 Drops of Pine Needle Oil

1 Drop of Wintergreen Oil

Directions:

Add these oils to your diffuser and enjoy.

26. Gingerbread Man Diffuser Recipe

3 Drops of Cinnamon Cassia Oil

2 Drops of Vanilla Oil

2 Drops of Ginger Oil

1 Drop of Clove Oil

1 Drop of Nutmeg Oil

Directions:

Add these oils to your diffuser and enjoy.

27. Holiday Eggnog Diffuser Recipe

10 Drops of Vanilla Oil

2 Drops of Nutmeg Oil

1 Drop of Cinnamon Cassia Oil

Directions:

Add these oils to your diffuser and enjoy.

28. Jolly Holly Holidays Diffuser Recipe

4 Drops of Lemon Oil

2 Drops of Cinnamon Cassia Oil

2 Drops of Ginger Oil

2 Drops of Nutmeg Oil

1 Drop of Clove Oil

Directions:

Add these oils to your diffuser and enjoy.

29. It's Christmas Again Diffuser Recipe

30 Drops of Pine Needle Oil

8 Drops of Atlas Cedar Oil

3 Drops of Cypress Oil

1 Drop of Orange Oil

Directions:

Add these oils to your diffuser and enjoy.

30. Under The Mistletoe Diffuser Recipe

5 Drops of Balsam Fir Needle Oil

2 Drops of Atlas Cedar Oil

1 Drop of Juniper Berry Oil

Directions:

Add these oils to your diffuser and enjoy.

31. Hearts & Mistletoe Diffuser Recipe

3 Drops of Pine Needle Oil

2 Drops of Atlas Cedar Oil

2 Drops of Rosemary Oil

1 Drop of Ylang Ylang Oil

1 Drop of Juniper Berry Oil

1 Drop of Eucalyptus Globulus Oil

Directions:

Add these oils to your diffuser and enjoy.

32. Santa's Sugar Cookies Diffuser Recipe

24 Drops of Vanilla Oil

2 Drops of Tangerine Oil

2 Drops of Cinnamon Bark Oil

1 Drop of Ginger Oil

Directions:

Add these oils to your diffuser and enjoy.

33. The Orchard Diffuser Recipe

12 Drops of Orange Oil

6 Drops of Patchouli Oil

4 Drops of Ginger Oil

Directions:

Add these oils to your diffuser and enjoy.

34. Fall Bouquet Diffuser Recipe

12 Drops of Orange Oil

3 Drops of Clove Oil

3 Drops of Cinnamon Cassia Oil

2 Drops of Nutmeg Oil

Directions:

Add these oils to your diffuser and enjoy.

35. Winter Icicles Diffuser Recipes

3 Drops of Peppermint Oil

3 Drops of Pennyroyal Oil

2 Drops of Rosemary Oil

1 Drop of Tea Tree Oil

1 Drop of Eucalyptus Globulus Oil

Directions:

Add these oils to your diffuser and enjoy.

36. Welcoming Blend Diffuser Recipe

3 Drops of Rosemary Oil

3 Drops of Lemon Oil

3 Drops of Lavender Oil

Directions:

Add these oils to your diffuser and enjoy.

37. Bliss Blend Diffuser Recipe

3 Drops of Grapefruit Oil

3 Drops of Wild Orange Oil

2 Drops of Bergamot Oil

2 Drops of Lemon Oil

Directions:

Add these oils to your diffuser and enjoy.

38. Fresh Air Blend Diffuser Recipe

3 Drops of Lime Oil

3 Drops of Lemon Oil

3 Drops of Melaleuca Oil

Directions:

Add these oils to your diffuser and enjoy.

39. Clean Air Blend Diffuser Recipe

4 Drops of Vetiver Oil

3 Drops of Peppermint Oil

3 Drops of Lemon Oil

Directions:

Add these oils to your diffuser and enjoy.

40. Fresher Feel Diffuser Recipe

3 Drops of Lemon Oil

2 Drops of Lime Oil

2 Drops of Cilantro Oil

2 Drops of Melaleuca Oil

Directions:

Add these oils to your diffuser and enjoy.

41. Nice Air Diffuser Recipe

3 Drops of Lemon Oil

2 Drops of Cilantro Oil

2 Drops of White Fir Oil

2 Drops of Lime Oil

2 Drops of Melaleuca Oil

Directions:

Add these oils to your diffuser and enjoy.

42. Manly Musk Diffuser Recipe

3 Drops of Arborvitae Oil

3 Drops of Cypress Oil

3 Drops of Bergamot Oil

Directions:

Add these oils to your diffuser and enjoy.

Essential Oil Recipes for Skincare

In this section, I'll be going over recipes that are perfect for all different types of skincare. Try these out whenever the need arises. I use many of these on a consistent basis and have had great results over the years. I hope they serve you just as well.

1. Ringworm & Athlete's Foot Recipe

1 Teaspoon of Massage Oil Base

2 Drops of Tea Tree Oil

1 Drop of Lavender Oil

Directions:

Add your drops to 1 teaspoon of your massage oil base. Can also use any carrier oil. Gently stir together to mix and apply using cotton swabs.

2. Minor Burns Recipe

2 Drops of Lavender Oil

Directions:

Apply ice-cold water immediately to your burn for approximately 10 minutes. Then apply 2 drops of your lavender lightly diluted.

3. Honey & Orange Body Wash Recipe

2/3 Cup of Castille Soap

1/4 Cup of Honey

2 Teaspoons of Sweet Almond Oil

2 Teaspoons of Vegetable Glycerin

1 Teaspoon of Vitamin E

40 to 50 drops of Orange Essential Oil

Directions:

Stir together all your ingredients. Add to a plastic pump bottle. Place in your shower and pump out whenever needed.

4. Lavender & Oatmeal Body Wash Recipe

3 Cups of Water

1/4 Cup of Liquid Castille Soap

1 Teaspoon of Vitamin E

1/4 Cup of Oatmeal

6 to 12 Drops of Lavender Oil

2 Teaspoons of Jojoba Oil

Directions:

Bring your 3 cups of water to a boil. Place your oatmeal in a glass bowl and pour your boiling water over your oatmeal. Allow to sit for between 1 to 2 hours and then strain your water to remove any oats from the water. Set to the side and discard your oats. Mix together all your other ingredients in a separate small-sized bowl. Pour in enough of your oil mixture to fill approximately 10% to 15% of your soap dispenser. Pour your water infused with oatmeal into the dispenser until almost full. Place lid back on dispenser. May have enough for two soap dispensers.

5. At Home Moisturizer Recipe

1/4 Cup of Coconut Oil

12 Drops of Lavender Oil

12 Drops of Orange Oil

12 Drops of Melrose Oil

8 Drops of Ylang Ylang Oil

Directions:

1. Add your coconut oil to a small-sized glass storage container. Add your essential oils and stir together until blended well together. Apply a pea-sized portion to your face each morning and evening.

6. Homemade Face Wash Recipe

2/3 Cup of Rose Water

1 Teaspoon of Liquid Carrier Oil

1/3 Cup of Castille Soap

4 Drops of Vitamin E

1/4 Teaspoon of Vegetable Glycerin

10 Drops of Chamomile Oil

10 Drops of Lavender Oil

5 Drops of Frankincense Oil

Directions:

Mix together all your ingredients in a glass pump bottle. Always give a gentle shake before using it.

7. Homemade Shower Gel Recipe

2/3 Cup of Castille Soap

1 Teaspoon of Vitamin E

2 Tablespoons of Raw Honey

2 Teaspoons of Vegetable Glycerin

1 Teaspoon of Jojoba Oil

10 Drops of Ylang Ylang Oil

5 Drops of Idaho Blue Spruce Oil

Directions:

Mix together all of your ingredients until they are well combined. Fill your 8 ounce mason jar and top it with your soap pump lid.

8. Twist of Peppermint Body Scrub Recipe

1/2 Cup of Organic Brown Sugar

1 Cup of Organic Coconut Oil

1/2 Cup of Organic Granulated White Sugar

3 Teaspoons of Organic Vanilla Extract

3 Teaspoons of Organic Coffee Grounds

2 Teaspoons of Organic Honey

1 Teaspoon of Peppermint Oil

Directions:

In a large sized bowl, combine all your ingredients and mix until well combined. Place inside an airtight container. Store in a cool place and allow the ingredients to become solid.

9. Minty Lemon Sugar Scrub Recipe

1 1/4 Cups of Granulated Sugar

1/2 Cup of Coconut Oil

1 Tablespoon of Lemon Juice

Zest of 1/2 Lemon

5 Drops of Lemon Oil

5 Drops of Peppermint Oil

Directions:

Mix all the ingredients together in a bowl. Store in the jar of your choice.

10. Foot Bath Detox Recipe

2 Cups of Epsom Salt

1 Tablespoon of Ground Ginger

5 Drops of Lavender Oil

5 Drops of Citrus Oil

1 Pint Sized Mason Jar

Directions:

Mix together all your ingredients in a medium-sized bowl. Pour them into your mason jar and secure the lid.

11. Whipped Body Butter Recipe

1/4 Cup of Raw Shea Butter

1/4 Cup of Coconut Oil

2 Ounces of Sweet Almond Oil

20 Drops of Desired Essential Oil

Directions:

Heat a saucepan over a low heat. Melt all your ingredients together until they completely liquefy. Pour into your stainless steel bowl and then place in the fridge overnight. Once it has harden back up, whip it for a few minutes using your mixer until it is all fluffy and light. Should have the consistency of cake icing.

12. DIY Anti-Aging Skin Butter Recipe

1 Cup of Coconut Oil (Must Be Solid)

10 Drops of Frankincense

10 Drops of Myrrh

Directions:

Scoop out your solid coconut oil into your bowl. Using a mixer of your choice, whip it at a high speed for approximately 5 minutes until it's light and airy. Add in your essential oils and whip again until well blended. Store in the jar of your choice.

13. Easy Hand Lotion Recipe

1/2 Cup Of Sweet Almond Oil

1/4 Cup of Beeswax

1/4 Cup of Coconut Oil

1 Tablespoon of Shea Butter

1 Teaspoon of Vitamin E Oil

20 Drops of Lavender Oil

Directions:

Place all of your ingredients except the lavender oil into a heavy canning jar. Place your jar into your saucepan and add enough water so the water level will come past your ingredients in the jar. Do not place any water in the jar itself. Place the lid on loosely so a little bit of air can get out. Heat your water over a medium heat and let the ingredients inside the jar melt. Should take approximately 20 minutes. Remove from heat and place your jar on a heat proof surface. Allow to cool for a couple of minutes. Add your lavender oil and stir gently to combine. Pour into a jar for storage. Should last approximately 6 months.

14. DIY Shaving Cream Recipe

1/2 Cup of Shea Butter

1/2 Cup of Organic Virgin Coconut Oil

1/3 Cup of Almond Oil

1 Tablespoon of Vitamin E Oil

10 Drops of Eucalyptus Oil

10 Drops of Peppermint Oil

Directions:

In your saucepan melt your shea butter and coconut oil. Take off the heat and add your vitamin E oil and almond oil. Place in your refrigerator until nearly solid. Add your peppermint and eucalyptus oil. Mix together with a mixer until well blended and fluffy. Place in glass containers for storage.

15. Remove Impurity Face Mask Recipe

2 Tablespoons of Bentonite Clay

4 Teaspoons of Aloe Vera

3 Capsules of Activated Charcoal

1 1/2 Ounces of Camomile Tea

2 Teaspoons of Shea Butter

1 Drop of Eucalyptus Oil

1 Drop of Peppermint Oil

Directions:

Start by brewing your tea and melting your shea butter using a double boiler. Once your tea is ready and your shea butter has been melted completely, mix them both together. Mix your bentonite clay and your activated charcoal. Add your clay mix to the tea mix and stir together. Add your aloe vera, eucalyptus oil, and peppermint oil. Mix together well. Store in an airtight container. When using be sure to apply all over your face and keep it on for approximately 15 minutes before washing it off.

16. Peppermint Chocolate Lip Balm Recipe

5 Tablespoons of Coconut Oil

1/4 Teaspoon of Cocoa Powder

3 Tablespoons of Beeswax

12 Drops of Peppermint Oil

Directions:

Melt your coconut oil and your beeswax in a glass measuring cup in your microwave. Once it is clear, stir in your cocoa powder and peppermint oil. Pour the mixture into empty lip balm tubes. Place in a cool area and allow to rest for several hours before using.

17. Brown Sugar Peppermint Lip Scrub Recipe

4 Tablespoons of Brown Sugar

3 Tablespoons of Organic Coconut Oil

2 Tablespoons of Honey

4 Drops of Peppermint Oil

Directions:

Mix together all your ingredients in a small-sized bowl. Store in a glass container.

18. Lemon Lip Balm Recipe

6 Tablespoons of Sweet Almond Oil

4 Tablespoons of Coconut Oil

4 Tablespoons of White Beeswax Pellets

10 Drops of Lemon Oil

Directions:

Fill a medium-sized sauce pot halfway with water and boil. Add your almond oil, coconut oil, and beeswax to a mason jar. Once your water is boiling, using a jar lifter, set your mason jar into the boiling water. As your jar get hot, the ingredients inside will begin to melt. Stir everything together inside your jar. Once the mixture is melted and clear, use your jar lifter to remove the jar from the heat. Stir in your lemon oil. Allow to cool. Once you can handle the mason jar safely, pour your liquid lip balm into empty lip balm containers. Place in a cool area and allow to solidify before using.

19. Homemade Mascara Recipe

1/4 Teaspoon of Bentonite Clay

1/4 Teaspoon of Black Mineral Powder

1/4 Teaspoon of Aloe Vera Gel

1/8 Teaspoon of Vegetable Glycerine

5 Drops of Lavender Oil

Directions:

Mix together all your ingredients in a small-sized bowl until smooth. If needed add more aloe gel until smooth. Use a spatula to scoop your mixture into your medicine dropper and slowly squirt your mixture into your mascara container.

20. Green Tea Eye Cream Recipe

2 Tablespoons of Almond Oil

1 Tablespoon of Shea Butter

3/4 Teaspoon of Beeswax

1 Bag of Green Tea

2 Drops of Vitamin E Oil

5 Drops of Peppermint Oil

Directions:

Melt your almond oil, vitamin E, beeswax, and shea butter in your double boiler. Once melted, open your green tea bag and pour into your melted oils. Allow the tea to seep for approximately 20 minutes over a low heat on your double boiler. Pour into strainer to remove any green tea bits. Mix in your peppermint oil. Pour into a container with a tight lid. Allow it to rest and reach room temperature before using. Should take a few hours.

21. Eye Makeup Remover Recipe

Baby Mild Castille Soap

2 Tablespoons of Jojoba Oil

1 Drop of Lavender Oil

Mix your lavender and jojoba oil. Fill up a bottle half way with your soap. Fill the remaining half with filtered water. Leave a little room at top for your oil mixture. Pour in oil mixture to bottle, add the lid tightly and shake it to mix.

22. Simple Homemade Shaving Cream Recipe

2 Tablespoons of V-6 Vegetable Oil Complex

2 Teaspoons of Lavender Mist Conditioner

2 Drops of Lavender Oil

2 Drops of Cedarwood Oil

1 Drop of Lime Oil

Directions:

Mix your lavender, lime, and cedarwood oils in your bowl. Add your V-6 and stir. Add your conditioner and whip it until the mixture is creamy and light.

23. Homemade Deodorant Recipe

1/4 Cup of Cornstarch

1/4 Cup of Baking Soda

1/4 Cup of Coconut Oil

20 Drops of Essential Oil of Your Choice

Directions:

Mix your ingredients together. Pack into your deodorant containers. You can use a big spoon to pour in your mixture and then pack it down regularly. Smooth off the tops using your hand.

24. Natural Skin Cream Recipe

1/2 Cup of Coconut Oil

20 Drops of Lavender Oil

5 Drops of Melaleuca Oil

Directions:

Mix all your ingredients together. Place into a glass container that can be closed.

25. Varicose Vein Body Butter Recipe

1/2 Cup of Organic Raw Shea Butter

1/4 Cup of Organic Cold Pressed Jojoba Oil

1/4 Cup of Organic Cold Pressed Coconut Oil

1 Tablespoon of Vitamin E

10 Drops of Cypress

10 Drops of Lemon

5 Drops of Helichrysum

5 Drops of Fennel

Directions:

Heat your coconut oil and shea butter in your double boiler on a medium low heat. Stir until your oil melts. Should take a few minutes. Remove from the heat. Add your jojoba oil, essential oils, and vitamin E. Place in your refrigerator for approximately 2 hours. Mix using a hand mixer for approximately 10 minutes until you've formed soft white peaks. Keep stored in a glass container. Good for approximately 6 months stored at room temperature. Can store in the fridge if you like cold body butter.

26. Homemade Stretch Mark Cream Recipe

1 Cup of Organic Unrefined Coconut Oil

1 Tablespoon of Vitamin E Oil

15 Drops of Frankincense Oil

15 Drops of Lavender Oil

Directions:

Combine all of your ingredients and beat for approximately 5 minutes using an electric mixer. Your consistency will be whipped and look like lotion. Store in a 1/2 pint mason jar.

27. Whipped Coconut Oil Cellulite Cream Recipe

1 Cup of Pure Organic Coconut Oil

15 Drops of Young Living Lemon Oil

5 Drops of Young Living Peppermint Oil

Directions:

In your glass bowl, combine coconut oil with your essential oils. Mix together well using your metal whisk until your mixture has a whipped appearance.

28. Perfect Skin Body Butter Recipe

2 ounces of Shea Butter

2 ounces of Evening Primrose Oil

10 Drops of Young Living Jasmine Oil

10 Drops of Young Living Frankincense Oil

Directions:

In your double boiler, melt your shea butter until it is a liquid (but let it get hot!). Before you add your evening primrose oil, make sure that your shea butter isn't hot. It should be room temperature or slightly warmer. Add your evening primrose oil and blend well using a hand mixer with a whisk attachment. Place your mixture in your fridge for a few minutes until it is cool but not solidified. Remove from your fridge, use a hand mixer on high speed to whip your oils into a white colored cream. It should turn into the texture similar to that of pancake batter. Add your essential oils, and mix on a low speed with a hand mixer until they are well-combined. Pour into glass containers with lids. The mixture will set and become the texture of butter.

29. Troubled Skin Treatment Recipe

3 Tablespoons of Rose Hip Seed Oil

1 Drop of Yarrow

1 Drop of Myrtle

1 Drop of Tea Tree

1 Drop of Lavender

Directions:

Mix all your ingredients together and apply topically as needed.

30. Regenerative Skin Blend Recipe

15 ML of Rose Hip Seed Oil & Tamanu Oil (50/ 50 Mix)

12 Drops of Helichrysum Italicum Oil

6 Drops of Rosemary Verbenone Oil

6 Drops of Carrot Seed Oil

Directions:

Mix all your ingredients together and apply topically as needed.

31. Scalp & Hair Recipe

30 ML of Jojoba Oil

8 Drops of Rosemary Oil

4 Drops of Peppermint Oil

4 Drops of Cypress

4 Drops of Lavender

Directions:

Mix all your ingredients together and apply topically as needed.

32. Oily Skin Treatment Recipe

1 Tablespoon of Coconut Butter

6 Drops of Tea Tree Oil

6 Drops of Lavender

2 Drops of Yarrow

Directions:

Mix all your ingredients together and apply topically as needed.

33. Dry Skin Assistance Recipe

15 ML of Argan

8 Drops of Rose Oil

4 Drops of Vetiver Oil

4 Drops of Sandalwood Oil

Directions:

Mix all your ingredients together and apply topically as needed.

34. Leg Circulation Recipe

1/2 Ounce of Carrier Oil

2 Drops of Chamomile

2 Drops of Geranium

2 Drops of Cypress

2 Drops of Yarrow

Directions:

Mix all your ingredients together and dot on affected areas as needed.

35. Rough Heels & Feet Blend Recipe

15 ML of Jojoba Oil

6 Drops of German Chamomile Oil

6 Drops of Carrot Seed Oil

3 Drops of Tagetes Oil

Directions:

Mix all your ingredients together and apply before bedtime as needed.

36. Clearer Nails Blend Recipe

30 ML of Jojoba Oil

8 Drops of Tea Tree Oil

4 Drops of Myrrh Oil

4 Drops of Tagetes Oil

Directions:

Mix all your ingredients together and apply topically to any affected areas.

37. Better Skin Blend Recipe

1 Ounce of Jojoba

7 Drops of Cypress Oil

5 Drops of Geranium

2 Drops of Cape Chamomile

Directions:

Mix all your ingredients together and apply topically as needed.

38. Younger Skin Assist Recipe

1 Tablespoon of Rose Hip Seed Oil

3 Drops of Tea Tree Oil

3 Drops of Lavender

2 Drops of Yarrow

2 Drops of Myrtle

Directions:

Mix all your ingredients together and apply topically as needed.

39. Mature Skin Assist Recipe

1 Ounce of Rose Hip Seed Oil

7 Drops of Cistus Oil

4 Drops of Frankincense / Myrrh Oil Distillation

4 Drops of Helichrysum Oil

2 Drops of Chamomile

Directions:

Mix all your ingredients together and apply topically as needed.

40. Stretch Mark Help Recipe

15 ML Rose Hip Seed Oil & Tamanu Oil (50/50 Mix)

10 Drops of Helichrysum Oil

6 Drops of Clementine Oil

3 Drops of Neroli Oil

3 Drops of Lavender Oil

Directions:

Mix all your ingredients together and apply topically as needed. Avoid direct sunlight once applied.

41. Clear Toenail Soak Recipe

6 Drops of Palmarosa Oil

3 Drops of Patchouli Oil

3 Drops of Lemongrass Oil

2 Drops of Tea Tree Oil

Directions:

Mix all your ingredients together and add to a warm foot bath.

42. Facial Toner Mist Recipe

2 Ounces of Rose Hydrosol

4 Drops of Yarrow Oil

4 Drops of Patchouli Oil

2 Drops of Cypress Oil

2 Drops Sandalwood Oil

Directions:

Mix all your ingredients together and apply as needed.

43. Injured Skin Treatment Recipe

1 Ounce of Rose Hip Seed Oil

3 Drops of St. John's Wort

3 Drops of Helichrysum Oil

2 Drops of Roman Chamomile Oil

Directions:

Mix all your ingredients together and apply topically as needed. Avoid direct sunlight once applied.

44. Repair Your Skin Blend Recipe

15 ML of Aloe Vera Gel

4 Drops of Helichrysum Oil

4 Drops of Lavender Oil

2 Drops of Rose Oil

Directions:

Mix all your ingredients together and apply topically as needed.

45. Facial Revitalizing Blend Recipe

15 ML of Jojoba Oil

5 Drops of Vitamin E Oil

8 Drops of Wild Carrot Seed

4 Drops of Helichrysum Italicum Oil

2 Drops of Frankincense Oil

2 Drops of Sandalwood Oil

Directions:

Mix all your ingredients together and apply topically as needed.

46. Combination Skin Cream Recipe

1/2 Ounce of Facial Moisturizer

3 Drops of Geranium Oil

3 Drops of Ylang Ylang Oil

Directions:

Mix all your ingredients together and apply on areas as needed.

47. Acne Away Recipe

30 ML of Borage Seed Oil

8 Drops of Lavender Oil

7 Drops of Tea Tree Oil

2 Drops of Chamomile Oil

2 Drops of Geranium Oil

2 Drops of Juniper Oil

Directions:

Mix all your ingredients together and apply sparingly on areas as needed twice each day for six weeks. If no results try increasing the concentration of the tea tree oil and lavender oil by a few drops.

48. Dermatitis Remedy Recipe

3 Drops of Frankincense Oil

2 Drops of Orange Oil

1 Drop of Tea Tree Oil

Directions:

Mix all your ingredients together and apply onto a tissue. Rub tissue over the affected areas as needed for a few minutes.

49. Jaundice Remedy Recipe

1 Tablespoon of Extra Virgin Olive Oil

2 Drops of Geranium Oil

2 Drops of Rosemary Oil

1 Drop of Lemon Oil

Directions:

Mix all your ingredients together. Massage mixture onto affected areas as needed.

50. Bad Make-Up Reaction Recipe

1 Tablespoon of Coconut Oil

3 Drops of Rose Oil

2 Drops of Bergamot Oil

1 Drop of Orange Oil

Directions:

Mix all your ingredients together. Massage mixture onto affected areas of your face. Do not get into your eyes, nose or mouth.

51. Better Nail Growth Recipe

1 Tablespoon of Coconut Oil

1 Drop of Rose Oil

1 Drop of Lavender Oil

Directions:

Mix all your ingredients together. Apply mixture to your bare nails on a daily basis

52. Skin Inflammation Recipe

1 Tablespoon of Coconut Oil

3 Drops of Frankincense Oil

2 Drops of Rosewood Oil

Directions:

Mix all your ingredients together. Dab onto a cotton ball and apply to your affected area as needed.

53. Sores Relief Recipe

1 Tablespoon of Coconut Oil

3 Drops of Lavender Oil

3 Drops of Rosewood Oil

Directions:

Mix all your ingredients together. Gently massage your mixture into your sores. Do this daily until the sores are healed.

54. Relieve Sunburn Recipe

1 Tablespoon of Avocado Oil

1 Drop of Eucalyptus Oil

1 Drop of Peppermint Oil

Directions:

Mix all your ingredients together. Apply mixture to your affected areas until healed.

55. Dry Skin Day Cream Recipe

80 ML of Aqueous Cream

10 ML of Rose Hip Oil

10 ML of Aloe Vera Gel

10 Drops of Palmarosa Oil

5 Drops of Sandalwood Oil

5 Drops of Geranium Oil

5 Drops of Lavender Oil

5 Drops of Jasmine Oil

Directions:

Mix all your ingredients together. Clean skin and pat dry. Apply your mixture.

56. Night Moisturizer Treatment Recipe

80 ML of Rose Hip Oil

5 Drops of Neroli Oil

5 Drops of Sandalwood Oil

5 Drops of Lavender Oil

5 Drops of Rose Oil

Directions:

Mix all your ingredients together. Clean face and pat dry. Apply your mixture.

57. Overnight Healing Treatment Recipe

100 ML of Rose Hip Oil

10 ML of Avocado Oil

5 Drops of Geranium Oil

5 Drops of Rose Oil

5 Drops of Sandalwood Oil

5 Drops of Lavender Oil

5 Drops of Neroli Oil

Directions:

Mix all your ingredients together. Clean face and pat dry. Place 1 dot of mixture on each cheek and dab it in. Place another 2 dots of mixture to cover your temples and forehead. Place another 3 dots on your neck. Place another dot on the back of each of your hands. Place a warm washcloth over your face. Relax for 10 minutes. Remove any mixture and dab your skin dry.

58. Oily Skin Steam Treatment Recipe

2 Drops of Lavender Oil

2 Drops of Juniper Oil

Directions:

Mix your ingredients together. Add your mixture to steaming water. Place a towel over your head and place head over the bowl. Be sure to keep eyes closed. After 5 minutes remove towel and wash off face of any debris.

59. Cleaner Pores Steam Treatment Recipe

2 Drops of Tea Tree Oil

2 Drops of Lemon Oil

Directions:

Mix your ingredients together. Add your mixture to steaming water. Place a towel over your head and place head over the bowl. Be sure to keep eyes closed. After 5 minutes remove towel and wash off face of any debris.

60. Acne Mask Recipe

25 ML of Clay Paste (Water mixed with clay)

2 Drops of Rose Oil

2 Drops of Bergamot Oil

2 Drops of Tea Tree Oil

Directions:

Mix all your ingredients together. Apply mixture to your face for approximately 15 minutes before washing off.

61. Oily Hair Conditioner Recipe

25ML of Olive Oil (Warmed up slightly)

5 Drops of Lavender Oil

5 Drops of Rosemary Oil

Directions:

Mix your ingredients together. Apply the mixture to your scalp and massage it in. Wrap your head in a cling wrap for approximately 20 minutes before rinsing mixture out.

62. Dry Hair Conditioner Recipe

25 ML of Jojoba Oil (Warmed up slightly)

5 Drops of Lavender Oil

5 Drops of Vetiver Oil

Directions:

Mix your ingredients together. Apply the mixture to your scalp and massage it in. Wrap your head in a cling wrap for approximately 20 minutes before rinsing mixture out.

63. Scalp Rub Treatment Recipe

5 Drops of Tea Tree Oil

5 Drops of Lavender Oil

Directions:

Mix your ingredients together. Apply the mixture to your scalp and massage it in.

Essential Oils Recipes for Colds & Flu & Congestion

In this section, I'll be going over recipes that are excellent for treating all different types of colds and flu. Try these out whenever you're feeling under the weather. I use many of these at least a few times a year and they always bring me great relief. I hope they do the same for you.

1. Sinus and Chest Congestion Recipe

2 Drops of Eucalyptus Oil

2 Drops of Tea Tree Oil

2 Drops of Lavender Oil

Directions:

Bring a pot of water to a boil and remove it from your stove. While it is still steaming add all of your drops. Cover your bowl and head using a towel and inhale for approximately 3 to 5 minutes while keeping your eyes closed at all times.

2. Common Cold Recipe

2 Teaspoons of Cream or Milk

2 Drops of Eucalyptus Oil

2 Drops of Rosemary Oil

2 Drops of Lavender Oil

Directions:

Add all your drops to 2 teaspoons of cream or milk. Pour mixture into a warm bath and stir water. Get in and soak. Can also place in a diffuser to help diffuse mixture into your room.

3. Defeat Sinus Congestion Recipe

2 Drops of Tea Tree Oil

2 Drops of Peppermint Oil

2 Drops of Eucalyptus Oil

Directions:

Bring a pot of water to a boil and remove the pot from your stove. While still steaming, add all your drops. Cover your pot and head immediately with your towel. Inhale for approximately 3 minutes while keeping your eyes closed the entire time.

4. Cough Begone Recipe

2 Drops of Lavender Oil

2 Drops of Eucalyptus Oil

Directions:

Bring a pot of water to a boil and remove the pot from your stove. While still steaming, add all your drops. Cover your pot and head immediately with your towel. Inhale for approximately 3 minutes while keeping your eyes closed the entire time.

5. Cough Away Recipe

4 Teaspoons of Massage Base Oil

2 Drops of Lavender Oil

2 Drops of Eucalyptus Oil

Directions:

Add all your drops to your 4 teaspoons of massage base oil. Apply your mixture to your chest and throat. You'll have enough for several applications. Every 8 hours reapply as necessary.

6. Daytime Cold & Flu Relief Recipe

2 Drops of Tea Tree Oil

2 Drops of Peppermint Oil

2 Drops of Lavender Oil

2 Drops of Eucalyptus Oil

Directions:

Add all your drops to a steaming bowl of water. Allow the bowl to stand so that your steam diffuses into your room.

7. Nighttime Cold & Flu Relief Recipe

2 Drops of Tea Tree Oil

2 Drops of Lavender Oil

Directions:

Add all your drops to a steaming bowl of water. Allow the bowl to stand so that your steam diffuses into your room.

8. Breathing Easy Diffuser Recipe

5 Drops of Hyssop Oil

5 Drops of Eucalyptus Globulus Oil

1 Drop of Pine Needle Oil

1 Drop of Cedarwood Oil

Directions:

Add these oils to your diffuser and enjoy.

9. Open Airways Diffuser Recipe

6 Drops of Hyssop Oil

4 Drops of Lavender Oil

2 Drops of Peppermint Oil

Directions:

Add these oils to your diffuser and enjoy.

10. Feeling Refreshed Diffuser Recipe

3 Drops of Ginger Oil

3 Drops of Lemon Oil

3 Drops of Clary Sage Oil

Directions:

Add these oils to your diffuser and enjoy.

11. Spring Is Here Diffuser Recipe

10 Drops of Lemongrass Oil

5 Drops of Lemon Oil

1 Drop of Eucalyptus Globulus Oil

Directions:

Add these oils to your diffuser and enjoy.

12. Purifying Room Diffuser Recipe

10 Drops of Lemon Oil

1 Drop of Grapefruit Oil

1 Drop of Tea Tree Oil

Directions:

Add these oils to your diffuser and enjoy.

13. Winter Wellness Recipe

30 ML of Tamanu Oil

16 Drops of Ravensara Oil

6 Drops of Chamomile Oil

4 Drops of Lavender Oil

4 Drops of Geranium Oil

3 Drops of Melissa Oil

Directions:

Mix all your ingredients together and apply on areas as needed.

14. Open Breathing Recipe

1 ounce of Carrier Oil

4 Drops of Juniper Berry

4 Drops of Frankincense Oil

2 Drops of Eucalyptus Oil

Directions:

Mix all your ingredients together and apply topically on your chest as needed.

15. Breathing Easier Recipe

1/2 Ounce of Carrier Oil

4 Drops of Chamomile Oil

4 Drops of Eastern Hemlock Oil

2 Drops of Peppermint Oil

2 Drops of Eucalyptus Oil

Directions:

Mix all your ingredients together and rub on chest as needed.

16. Clear Breath Blend Diffuser Recipe

8 Drops of Ravensara Oil

3 Drops of Thyme Oil

3 Drops of Eucalyptus Oil

3 Drops of Oregano Oil

Directions:

Add these oils to your diffuser and enjoy.

17. Breathing Deeply Blend Recipe

30 ML of Jojoba Oil

8 Drops of Frankincense Oil

6 Drops of Eucalyptus Oil

3 Drops of Pine Oil

3 Drops of Rosemary Oil

2 Drops of Peppermint Oil

Directions:

Mix all your ingredients together and apply on areas as needed.

18. Winter Assistance Blend Diffuser Recipe

2 Drops of Marjoram Oil

2 Drops of Lemon Oil

2 Drops of Eucalyptus Smithii Oil

2 Drops of Pine Oil

1 Drop of Thyme Oil

1 Drop of Rosemary Oil

Directions:

Add these oils to your diffuser and enjoy.

19. Kid's Breathe Blend Recipe

1/2 Ounce of Carrier Oil

1 Drop of Lavender Oil

1 Drop of Silver Fir

Directions:

Mix all your ingredients together and rub on your chest before going to bed.

20. Cold & Flu Vapor Therapy Blend

2 Drops of Eucalyptus Smithii Oil

2 Drops of Marjoram Oil

2 Drops of Lemon Oil

2 Drops of Corsican Pine Oil

1 Drop of Thyme Oil

1 Drop of Rosemary Oil

Directions:

Mix all your ingredients together in steaming water and inhale with your head covered, slowly taking deeper and deeper breaths through both your mouth and nose. Keep your eyes closed at all times.

21. Gentle Lung Recipe

4 Drops of Eucalyptus Smithii Oil

4 Drops of Pinon Pine Oil

4 Drops of Desert Marjoram Oil

Directions:

Mix all your ingredients together. Add one drop to your cloth and inhale.

22. Clear Airways Recipe

1 Ounce of Carrier Oil

4 Drops of Frankincense Oil

4 Drops of Juniper Berry Oil

2 Drops of Cedar Oil

2 Drops of Eucalyptus Oil

Directions:

Mix all your ingredients together and rub on your chest as needed.

23. Immune Booster Diffuser Recipe

2 Drops of Wild Orange Oil

2 Drops of Cinnamon Oil

2 Drops of Eucalyptus Oil

2 Drops of Clove Oil

2 Drops of Rosemary Oil

Directions:

Add these oils to your diffuser and enjoy a healthier immune system.

24. Increased Immune System Diffuser Recipe

2 Drops of Lemon Oil

2 Drops of Eucalyptus Oil

1 Drop of Clove Oil

1 Drop of Lime Oil

1 Drop of Rosemary Oil

Directions:

Add these oils to your diffuser and enjoy a healthier immune system.

25. Respiratory Wellness Diffuser Recipe

2 Drops of Peppermint Oil

1 Drop of Eucalyptus Oil

1 Drop of Lemon Oil

1 Drop of Rosemary Oil

Directions:

Add these oils to your diffuser and enjoy better respiratory wellness.

26. Immune Spike Diffuser Recipe

1 Drop of Wild Orange Oil

1 Drop of Cinnamon Bark Oil

1 Drop of Eucalyptus Oil

1 Drop of Clove Oil

1 Drop of Rosemary Oil

Directions:

Add these oils to your diffuser and enjoy a healthier immune system.

27. Congested Chest Relief Recipe

1 Tablespoon of Extra Virgin Olive Oil

2 Drops of Niaouli Oil

1 Drop of Lavender Oil

1 Drop of Sweet Birch Oil

Directions:

Mix all your ingredients together and store in a dark colored bottle. Massage mixture onto your chest before bed as needed.

28. Pink Eye Remedy Recipe

1 Teaspoon of Coconut Oil

2 Drops of Lavender Oil

2 Drops of Tea Tree Oil

Directions:

Mix all your ingredients together. Apply around your eyes. Do not get in eyes. If any of the mixture gets into your eyes do not rinse them with water. Instead, rinse them with olive oil or coconut oil.

29. Persistent Cough Remedy Recipe

3 Tablespoons of Honey

2 Drops of Lemon Oil

1 Drop of Eucalyptus Oil

1 Drop of Peppermint Oil

Directions:

Mix all your ingredients together. Take them orally every three hours as needed.

30. Earache Relief Recipe

1 Tablespoon of Jojoba Oil

2 Drops of Roman Chamomile Oil

2 Drops of Sandalwood Oil

Directions:

Mix all your ingredients together. Place 2 to 3 drops in the affected ear 3 times a day as needed.

31. Ear Infection Remedy Recipe

1 Tablespoon of Coconut Oil

2 Drops of Peppermint Oil

1 Drop of Rose Oil

1 Drop of Lavender Oil

Directions:

Mix all your ingredients together. Rub your mixture on the outside of your ears and down your neck to help treat any infection.

32. Flu Reliever Recipe

1 Tablespoon of Grape Seed Oil

2 Drops of Geranium Oil

1 Drop of Sandalwood Oil

1 Drop of Lemon Oil

Directions:

Mix all your ingredients together and shake well. Apply mixture to the sides of the nose and underneath your jawline.

33. Influenza Relief Recipe

500 ML of Boiling Water

2 Drops of Eucalyptus Oil

1 Drop of Sandalwood Oil

1 Drop of Lavender Oil

1 Drop of Lemon Oil

Directions:

Add all your ingredients to the boiling water. Pour into a steam basin. Place your head over the basin and cover using a towel. Inhale deeply. Do this twice a day until symptoms are gone.

34. Relieve Nasal Congestion Recipe

3 Drops of Sweet Orange Oil

2 Drops of Lemon Oil

1 Blank Inhaler

Directions:

Mix all your ingredients together. Add to your inhaler and inhale deeply several times as needed.

35. Infection Begone Recipe

250 ML of Epsom Salts

125 ML of Baking Soda

125 ML of Milk

2 Drops of Sweet Orange Oil

2 Drops of Juniper Berry Oil

2 Drops of Eucalyptus Oil

Directions:

Draw a hot bath. Run your baking soda and Epsom salt under the bath water so it gets dissolved. Mix your essential oils and milk together. Add your mixture to the bath. Soak for approximately 30 minutes.

36. Flu Beater Treatment Recipe

80 ML of Sweet Almond Oil

3 Drops of Mandarin Oil

3 Drops of Tea Tree Oil

3 Drops of Eucalyptus Oil

Directions:

Mix all your ingredients together. Massage mixture into your feet, chest, and back. Use this immediately before bedtime.

37. Flu Diffuser Blend Recipe

2 Drops of Lavender Oil

2 Drops of Eucalyptus Oil

2 Drops of Tea Tree Oil

Directions:

Add these oils to your diffuser before going to bed.

38. Fever Remover Recipe

1 Drop of Eucalyptus Oil

1 Drop of Tea Tree Oil

1 Drop of Peppermint Oil

Directions:

Draw a lukewarm bath. Add your oils to the bath. Soak in the mixture until feeling less feverish or you feel cold chills.

39. Fever Foot Rub Recipe

60 ML of Sweet Almond Oil

2 Drops of Tea Tree Oil

2 Drops of Lemon Oil

2 Drops of Eucalyptus Oil

Directions:

Mix all your ingredients together. Gently massage the mixture into the soles of each foot. Rub a small amount of the mixture onto your back and chest. Apply 3 times a day as needed.

Essential Oils Recipes for Aches, Pains, & Common Ailments

In this section, I'll be discussing recipes that will help to ease all different types of aches, pains, and common ailments. The older I get the more I find use for these recipes. Give these a try whenever the need arises. Hopefully, you'll find these recipes as helpful as I have over the years.

1. Muscle Pain Recipe

4 Teaspoons of Massage Oil Base

2 Drops of Rosemary Oil

2 Drops of Lavender Oil

Directions:

Add your drops to 4 teaspoons of your massage oil base. Can also use any carrier oil or plain base. Stir together and gently massage on your body in the affected areas.

2. Headache Relief Recipe

2 Drops of Lavender Oil

Directions:

Simply massage 2 drops of lavender (undiluted) on the base of your skull and into your temples.

3. Pre-Sports Rub Recipe

4 Teaspoons of Massage Oil Base

2 Drops of Rosemary Oil

1 Drop of Eucalyptus Oil

1 Drop of Lavender Oil

Directions:

Blend together all of your essential oils. Add 4 teaspoons of your massage oil base. Gently stir them to mix and apply to your body before beginning to exercise.

4. Post-Sports Rub Recipe

4 Teaspoons of Massage Oil Base

2 Drops of Lavender Oil

1 Drop of Rosemary Oil

1 Drop of Juniper Oil

Directions:

Blend together all of your essential oils. Add 4 teaspoons of your massage oil base. Gently stir them to mix and apply to your body after finishing your exercises.

5. After Impact Recipe

8 Drops of German Chamomile Oil

8 Drops of Helichrysum Italicum Oil

Directions:

Mix all your ingredients together and apply as needed.

6. Cooling Body Blend Recipe

2 Teaspoons of Chamomile Hydrosol

1 Tablespoon of Lavender Hydrosol

2 Ounces of Aloe Vera Gel

6 Drops of Helichrysum Oil

5 Drops of Lavender Oil

3 Drops of Chamomile Oil

Directions:

Mix all your ingredients together. Shake container and apply to areas of your body that feel heat discomfort.

7. After Workout Massage Recipe

15 ML of Jojoba Oil

4 Drops of Frankincense Oil

4 Drops of Black Pepper Oil

2 Drops of Clary Sage Oil

1 Drop of Peppermint Oil

Directions:

Mix all your ingredients together and apply as needed.

8. Cerebral Circulation Formula Recipe

15 ML of Jojoba Oil

5 Drops of Ginger Grass Oil

4 Drops of Frankincense

1 Drop of Peppermint Oil

Directions:

Mix all your ingredients together and apply to the head and back of your neck as needed.

9. Water Balance Blend Recipe

15 ML Jojoba Oil

4 Drops of Lentisque Oil

4 Drops of Juniper Berry Oil

4 Drops of Geranium Oil

4 Drops of Cypress Oil

4 Drops of Rosemary Oil

2 Drops of Lavender Oil

Directions:

Mix all your ingredients together and apply as needed.

10. Minor Ouch Blend Recipe

30 ML of Jojoba Oil

4 Drops of German Chamomile Oil

4 Drops of Helichrysum Oil

2 Drops of Silver Fir

2 Drops of Rosemary Oil

2 Drops of Cedar Oil

Directions:

Mix all your ingredients together and apply as needed.

11. Repetitive Work Wrist Assistance Recipe

1/2 Ounce of Carrier Oil

4 Drops of Marjoram Oil

3 Drops of Helichrysum Oil

2 Drops of Ginger Oil

2 Drops of Birch Oil

Directions:

Mix all your ingredients together and apply as needed.

12 Better Lymphatic Flow Recipe

2 Cups of Sea Salt

1 Cup of Jojoba Oil

8 Drops of Dwarf Jupiter Oil

7 Drops of Lentisque Oil

4 Drops of Rosemary Oil

Directions:

Mix all your ingredients together and apply as needed.

13. Healthier Joints Blend Recipe

15 ML of Jojoba Oil

8 Drops of Pinon Juniper Oil

4 Drops of Rosemary Oil

4 Drops of Eucalyptus Globulus Oil

4 Drops of Marjoram

2 Drops of Ginger Oil

Directions:

Mix all your ingredients together and apply as needed.

14. My Poor Muscles Recipe

15 ML of Jojoba Oil

10 Drops of Laurel Oil

7 Drops of Rosemary Oil

5 Drops of Birch Oil

5 Drops of Helichrysum Oil

Directions:

Mix all your ingredients together and apply as needed.

15. Warm Extremities Recipe

1/2 Ounce of Carrier Oil

3 Drops of Lemon Oil

3 Drops of Clove Oil

2 Drops of Cinnamon Oil

1 Drop of Eucalyptus Oil

1 Drop of Rosemary Oil

Directions:

Mix all your ingredients together and apply to the bottom of your feet as needed. Avoid direct exposure to sunlight after applying.

16. Women's Moon Comfort Recipe

30 ML of Jojoba Oil

6 Drops of Clary Sage Oil

4 Drops of Angelica Oil

4 Drops of Roman Chamomile Oil

4 Drops of Cardamom Oil

Directions:

Mix all your ingredients together and apply as needed.

17. Healthier Lymph Scrub Recipe

1 Cup of Fine Sea Salt

1/2 Cup of Jojoba Oil

12 Drops of Laurel Oil

7 Drops of Grapefruit Oil

Directions:

Mix all your ingredients together and apply as needed. Avoid direct exposure to sunlight after applying.

18. Sore Muscle Recipe

30 ML of Marula Oil

6 Drops of Eucalyptus Globulus Oil

6 Drops of Helichrysum Oil

4 Drops of Ginger Oil

2 Drops of Sweet Birch Oil

Directions:

Mix all your ingredients together and apply as needed.

19. Soothing Massage Recipe

15 ML of Jojoba Oil

6 Drops of Ginger Oil

4 Drops of Orange Oil

2 Drops of Neroli Oil

2 Drops of Black Pepper Oil

Directions:

Mix all your ingredients together and apply as needed. Avoid direct exposure to sunlight after applying.

20. Workout Aftermath Blend Recipe

30 ML of Marula Oil

6 Drops of Lavender Oil

4 Drops of Frankincense

4 Drops of Rosemary Oil

Directions:

Mix all your ingredients together and rub into joints and muscles as needed.

21. Comfort Massage Blend Recipe

30 ML of Jojoba Oil

4 Drops of German Chamomile Oil

4 Drops of Helichrysum Oil

2 Drops of Cedar Oil

2 Drops of Alpine Fir Oil

2 Drops of Rosemary Oil

Directions:

Mix all your ingredients together and massage into areas as needed.

22. Deeper Rest Recipe

30 ML of Jojoba Oil

4 Drops of Lavender Oil

2 Drops of Roman Chamomile Oil

1 Drop of Cedarwood Oil

Directions:

Mix all your ingredients together and apply as needed.

23. Ease Your Belly Blend Recipe

15 ML of Marula Oil

4 Drops of Fennel Oil

3 Drops of Peppermint Oil

2 Drops of Ginger Oil

1 Drop of Nutmeg Oil

Directions:

Mix all your ingredients together and apply over your abdomen as needed.

24. Gentle Aromatic Bath Recipe

1 Tablespoon of Honey

1 Drop of Rose Oil

Directions:

Add rose oil to honey and add mixture to your bath.

25. Purify Foot Soak Recipe

6 Drops of Palmarosa Oil

3 Drops of Patchouli Oil

3 Drops of Lemongrass Oil

2 Drops of Tea Tree Oil

Directions:

Mix all your ingredients together and add to warm water for a nice purifying foot bath.

26. Cooling Foot Bath Recipe

8 Drops of Juniper Berry Oil

4 Drops of Cypress Oil

4 Drops of Rosemary Oil

4 Drops of Rhododendron Oil

Directions:

Mix all your ingredients together and add to cool water for a healthy inflammation response.

27. Tummy Massage Recipe

15 ML of Marula Oil

4 Drops of Peppermint Oil

4 Drops of Grapefruit Oil

2 Drops of Fennel Oil

2 Drops of Ginger Oil

Directions:

Mix all your ingredients together and apply as needed. Avoid direct exposure to sunlight after applying.

28. Digestive Assistance Massage Recipe

15 ML of Marula Oil

4 Drops of Peppermint Oil

4 Drops of Grapefruit Oil

2 Drops of Fennel Oil

2 Drops of Ginger Oil

Directions:

Mix all your ingredients together and apply as needed. Avoid direct exposure to sunlight after applying.

29. Seasonal Discomfort Diffuser Recipe

3 Drops of Peppermint Oil

3 Drops of Lavender Oil

3 Drops of Lemon Oil

Directions:

Add these oils to your diffuser and enjoy relief.

30. Headache Relief Diffuser Recipe

2 Drops of Thyme Oil

2 Drops of Marjoram Oil

2 Drops of Lavender Oil

2 Drops of Peppermint Oil

2 Drops of Rosemary Oil

Directions:

Add these oils to your diffuser and enjoy relief.

31. Headache Eraser Diffuser Recipe

6 Drops of Peppermint Oil

4 Drops of Eucalyptus Oil

2 Drops of Myrrh Oil

Directions:

Add these oils to your diffuser and enjoy relief.

32. Headache Eliminator Diffuser Recipe

9 Drops of Rosemary Oil

5 Drops of Melaleuca Oil

4 Drops of Geranium Oil

3 Drops of Peppermint Oil

2 Drops of Lavender Oil

2 Drops of Eucalyptus Oil

Directions:

Add these oils to your diffuser and enjoy relief.

33. Better Blood Sugar Recipe

1 Tablespoon of Borage Seed Oil

3 Drops of Eucalyptus Oil

Directions:

Mix your ingredients together in a small-sized bowl. Massage your mixture onto the soles of your feet twice daily to help you regulate your blood sugar levels.

34. Bruises Begone! Recipe

1 Tablespoon of Sweet Almond Oil

1 Drop of Citronella Oil

1 Drop of Sandalwood Oil

1 Drop of Yarrow Oil

Directions:

Mix your ingredients together in a small-sized bowl. Massage onto the affected area as needed.

35. Anti-Bacterial Relief Recipe

3 Drops of Citronella Oil

2 Drops of Tea Tree Oil

1 Drop of Coconut Oil

1 Drop of Rosemary Oil

1 Drop of Lavender Oil

Directions:

Mix all your ingredients together and apply on areas of your body as needed.

36. Allergy Relief Recipe

3 Drops of Eucalyptus Oil

2 Drops of Sandalwood Oil

2 Drops of Rosemary Oil

1 Blank Inhaler

Directions:

Add all your ingredients to your blank inhaler and use inhaler whenever struck with allergy or hay fever attack.

37. Arthritis Ease Recipe

1 Tablespoon of Macadamia Nut Oil

2 Drops of Roman Chamomile Oil

1 Drop of Peppermint Oil

1 Drop of Eucalyptus Oil

1 Drop of Lavender Oil

Directions:

Mix all your ingredients together and massage on areas of your body as needed.

38. Improved Blood Circulation Recipe

1 Tablespoon of Primrose Oil

3 Drops of Marjoram Oil

2 Drops of Goldenrod Oil

1 Drop of Cypress Oil

Directions:

Mix all your ingredients together and apply on different parts of your body. I recommend the wrists, upper back, calves, and chest areas.

39. Asthma Relief Recipe

15 ML of Macadamia Nut Oil

6 Drops of Lavender Oil

3 Drops of Eucalyptus Oil

3 Drops of Rosemary Oil

1 Drop of Ginger Oil

Directions:

Mix all your ingredients together in a dark glass bottle. Shake well. Massage mixture onto your back and chest on a daily basis.

40. Heal Chapped Lips Recipe

1 Tablespoon of Coconut Oil

1 Drop of Rosewood Oil

1 Drop of Roman Chamomile Oil

Directions:

Mix all your ingredients together and apply on lips as many times as needed each day until your chapped lips are gone.

41. Croup Remedy Recipe

1 Tablespoon of Avocado Oil

2 Drops of Sandalwood Oil

2 Drops of Ravensara Oil

2 Drops of Marjoram Oil

1 Drop of Thyme Oil

Directions:

Mix all your ingredients together and massage onto your chest as needed.

42. Detoxify Yourself Diffuser Recipe

1 Tablespoon of Macadamia Nut Oil

3 Drops of Juniper Oil

Directions:

Mix all your ingredients together. Add this mixture to your diffuser in the room you spend the most time in.

43. Dust Allergy Diffuser Recipe

3 Drops of Melissa Oil

1 Drop of Basil Oil

1 Drop of Geranium Oil

Directions:

Mix all your ingredients together. Add this mixture to your diffuser in the room you spend the most time in.

44. Heat Rash Relief Recipe

1 Tablespoon of Borage Oil

3 Drops of Patchouli Oil

3 Drops of Neroli Oil

Directions:

Mix all your ingredients together. Massage mixture onto your rash as needed.

45. Constipation Relief Recipe

1 Tablespoon of Coconut Oil

1 Drop of Rosemary Oil

1 Drop of Orange Oil

1 Drop of Ginger Oil

Directions:

Mix all your ingredients together and store in a dark colored bottle. Massage mixture into your stomach in a clockwise direction.

46. Hay Fever Recipe

3 Drops of Frankincense Oil

3 Drops of Peppermint Oil

1 Blank Inhaler

Directions:

Mix all your essential oils together and add to your inhaler. Inhale deeply whenever you feel an attack coming on.

47. Heartache Relief

1 Tablespoon of Primrose Oil

3 Drops of Lavender Oil

2 Drops of Bergamot Oil

1 Drop of Tea Tree Oil

Directions:

Mix all your ingredients together. Massage mixture onto your chest as needed.

48. Indigestion Relief Recipe

1 Tablespoon of Coconut Oil

3 Drops of Grapeseed Oil

3 Drops of Lemongrass Oil

Directions:

Mix all your ingredients together and place them in a bottle. Inhale deeply as needed.

49. Ingrown Hair Recipe

3 Drops of Tea Tree Oil

3 Drops of Peppermint Oil

Plain Body Wash or Lotion

Directions:

Mix all your ingredients together. Shake the mixture and apply to your body as needed.

50. Intestinal Issues Recipe

5 ML of Vegetable Carrier Oil

2 Drops of Rosemary Oil

1 Drop of Clove Oil

1 Drop of Chamomile Oil

1 Drop of Peppermint Oil

Directions:

Mix all your ingredients together. Apply mixture over your stomach as needed.

51. Jaw Pain Relief

2 Tablespoons of Avocado Oil

3 Drops of Olbas Oil

1 Drop of Juniper Oil

Directions:

Mix all your ingredients together. Massage mixture into your jawline to loosen your jaw and relieve pain.

52. Overcome Nausea Recipe

3 Drops of Tarragon Oil

1 Blank Inhaler

Directions:

Add oil to your inhaler. Inhale deeply as needed.

53. Neck Strain Relief Recipe

1 Tablespoon of Avocado Oil

3 Drops of Lavender Oil

1 Drop of Rosemary Oil

Directions:

Mix all your ingredients together. Massage mixture into your strained neck area as needed.

54. Renal Function Remedy Recipe

1 Tablespoon of Coconut Oil

2 Drops of Ledum Oil

1 Drop of Celery Seed Oil

1 Drop of Carrot Seed Oil

Directions:

Mix all your ingredients together. Massage mixture gently into your sides where kidneys are located.

55. Shoulder Pain Relief Recipe

1 Tablespoon of Avocado Oil

3 Drops of Sandalwood Oil

1 Drop of German Chamomile Oil

Directions:

Mix all your ingredients together. Massage mixture gently into your shoulder area several times each day.

56. Aching Knees Recipe

1 Tablespoon of Avocado Oil

3 Drops of Ginger Oil

3 Drops of Sweet Orange Oil

Directions:

Mix all your ingredients together. Massage mixture into your knee as needed.

57. Aching Legs Recipe

1 Tablespoon of Coconut Oil

3 Drops of Marjoram Oil

2 Drops of Jasmine Oil

Directions:

Mix all your ingredients together. Massage mixture into your legs as needed.

58. Swollen Ankles Relief Recipe

1 Tablespoon of Avocado Oil

3 Drops of Ginger Oil

3 Drops of Peppermint Oil

Directions:

Mix all your ingredients together. Massage mixture into your ankles as needed.

59. Relieve Thrush Recipe

1 Tablespoon of Vegetable Oil

2 Drops of Rosewood Oil

1 Drop of Thyme Oil

1 Drop of Chamomile Oil

Directions:

Mix all your ingredients together. Apply mixture to the roof of your mouth.

60. Tonsillitis Relief Recipe

1 Tablespoon of Coconut Oil

2 Drops of Ginger Oil

2 Drops of Tea Tree Oil

1 Drop of Lemon Oil

1 Drop of Lavender Oil

1 Drop of Roman Chamomile Oil

Directions:

Mix all your ingredients together. Apply mixture to the outside area of your throat and gently massage.

61. Yeast Infection Recipe

3 Drops of Oregano Oil

2 Drops of Lavender Oil

Directions:

Mix all your ingredients together. Ingest the mixture twice a day until for up to 2 weeks until your infection is gone.

62. Immunity Tonic Mix Recipe

100 ML of Sweet Almond Oil

6 Drops of Bergamot Oil

6 Drops of Lavender Oil

3 Drops of Tea Tree Oil

3 Drops of Lemon Oil

2 Drops of Myrrh Oil

Directions:

Mix all your ingredients together. Massage mixture over areas of body that are prone to developing physical issues.

63. Immunity Booster Cream Recipe

50 ML of Aqueous Cream

2 Drops of Chamomile Oil

2 Drops of Lavender Oil

2 Drops of Marjoram Oil

Directions:

Mix all your ingredients together. Massage mixture into the soles of your feet each night for 2 weeks.

64. Improve Immunity Diffuser Blend Recipe

2 Drops of Lavender Oil

2 Drops of Tea Tree Oil

Directions:

Add oils to your diffuser and enjoy.

65. Pain Reliever Recipe

10 ML of Sweet Almond Oil

10 Ml of Jojoba Oil

2 Drops of Chamomile Oil

2 Drops of Sweet Marjoram Oil

2 Drops of Melissa Oil

Directions:

Mix all your ingredients together. Massage mixture into affected areas twice daily as needed.

66. Diaper Rash Treatment Recipe

250 ML Aqueous Cream

10 Drops of Lavender Oil

5 Drops of Palmarosa Oil

5 Drops of Geranium Oil

5 Drops of Sandalwood Oil

Directions:

Mix all your ingredients together. Apply mixture onto affected areas as needed.

67. Psoriasis Treatment Cream Recipe

200 ML of Thick Aqueous Cream

10 ML of Borage Oil

10 ML Avocado Oil

5 Drops of Tea Tree Oil

5 Drops of Myrrh Oil

5 Drops of Lavender Oil

Directions:

Mix all your ingredients together. Apply mixture onto affected areas as needed.

Essential Oils Relaxing Recipes

In this section, I'll be discussing recipes that will allow you to reach a state of ease and relaxation. I love using these whenever I've had a stressful day. If you need to find some calm and peace of mind these recipes will do the trick.

1. Relaxation Massage Oil Recipe

6 Teaspoons of Massage Oil Base

4 Drops of Lavender Oil

1 Drop of Frankincense Oil

1 Drop of Petitgrain Oil

Directions:

Add all your drops to 6 teaspoons of your massage oil base. Mix together. Add to your warm bath.

2. Rest & Calm Recipe

1 Teaspoon of Cream or Milk

4 Drops of Lavender Oil

Directions:

Add your drops to a teaspoon of your cream or milk. Stir together. Pour into your warm bath. Stir the bath water and soak.

3. Sleep Peacefully Recipe

1 Teaspoon of Cream or Milk

3 Drops of Lavender Oil

1 Drop of Clary Sage Oil

Directions:

Mix all your drops with a teaspoon of your cream or milk. Add to your warm bath and soak.

4. Stress Reliever Massage Oil Recipe

5 teaspoons of Massage Oil Base

2 Drops of Petitgrain Oil

2 Drops of Lavender Oil

1 Drop of Ylang Ylang Oil

Directions:

Add all your drops to 5 teaspoons of your massage oil base. Gently stir it all together and massage mixture into your body.

5. A Goodnight Rest Diffuser Recipe

4 Drops of Marjoram Oil

4 Drops of Lavender Oil

4 Drops of Cypress Oil

Directions:

Add these oils to your diffuser and enjoy.

6. Deep Sleep Diffuser Recipe

20 Drops of Neroli Oil

2 Drops of Sage Oil

1 Drop of Ylang Ylang Oil

Directions:

Add these oils to your diffuser and enjoy.

7. Sweet Peace Of Mind Diffuser Recipe

10 Drops of Lavender Oil

6 Drops of Chamomile Oil

Directions:

Add these oils to your diffuser and enjoy.

8. Nice & Relaxed Diffuser Recipe

15 Drops of Vanilla Oil

2 Drops of Lavender Oil

2 Drops of Jasmine Oil Blend

Directions:

Add these oils to your diffuser and enjoy.

9. Time to Unwind Diffuser Recipe

2 Drops of Sandalwood Oil Blend

2 Drops of Lavender Oil

1 Drop of Chamomile Oil

Directions:

Add these oils to your diffuser and enjoy.

10. Breathing Deep Diffuser Recipe

2 Drops of Rosemary Oil

2 Drops of Myrrh Oil

1 Drop of Eucalyptus Globulus Oil

Directions:

Add these oils to your diffuser and enjoy.

11. Calming Relaxer Diffuser Recipe

7 Drops of Lavender Oil

3 Drops of Geranium Oil

1 Drop of Chamomile Oil

Directions:

Add these oils to your diffuser and enjoy.

12. Sleepy Time Diffuser Recipe

3 Drops of Chamomile Oil

3 Drops of Juniper Berry Oil

3 Drops of Lavender Oil

Directions:

Add these oils to your diffuser and sleep better.

13. Sound Asleep Diffuser Recipe

4 Drops of Cedarwood Oil

3 Drops of Lavender Oil

Directions:

Add these oils to your diffuser and sleep better.

14. Lights Out Diffuser Recipe

3 Drops of Lavender Oil

3 Drops of Vetiver Oil

2 Drops of Frankincense Oil

Directions:

Add these oils to your diffuser and sleep better.

15. Fast Asleep Diffuser Recipe

3 Drops of Balance Oil

2 Drops of Vetiver Oil

2 Drops of Roman Chamomile Oil

2 Drops of Lavender Oil

Directions:

Add these oils to your diffuser and sleep better.

16. Sleeping Easy Diffuser Recipe

3 Drops of Lavender Oil

2 Drops of Marjoram Oil

1 Drop of Roman Chamomile Oil

1 Drop of Orange Oil

Directions:

Add these oils to your diffuser and sleep better.

17. Nighty Nite Diffuser Recipe

2 Drops of Vetiver Oil

2 Drops of Chamomile Oil

2 Drops of Lavender Oil

Directions:

Add these oils to your diffuser and sleep better.

18. Sayonara Stress Diffuser Recipe

2 Drops of Bergamot Oil

2 Drops of Frankincense Oil

Directions:

Add these oils to your diffuser and say goodbye to stress.

19. Chill Out Diffuser Recipe

2 Drops of Cedarwood Oil

2 Drops of Vetiver Oil

Directions:

Add these oils to your diffuser and relax.

Essential Oils Uplifting Recipes

In this section, I'm going to go over a few recipes that are good when you need to raise your spirits or need a boost to get going.

1. Uplift Daytime Recipe

6 Teaspoons of Massage Oil Base

2 Drops of Rosewood Oil

2 Drops of Geranium Oil

2 Drops of Bergamot Oil

Directions:

Add all your drops to your 6 teaspoons of massage oil. Mix together. Wear it as a fragrance, inhale from the bottle directly, or use as a gentle massage oil.

2. Uplift Nighttime Recipe

6 Teaspoons of Massage Oil Base

2 Drops of Ylang Ylang Oil

2 Drops of Bergamot Oil

2 Drops of HoWood Oil

Directions:

Add all your drops to your 6 teaspoons of massage oil. Mix together. Wear it as a fragrance, inhale from the bottle directly, or use as a gentle massage oil.

3. Fun In the Summer Diffuser Recipe

1 Drop of Lavender Oil

1 Drop of Grapefruit Oil

1 Drop of Peppermint Oil

Directions:

Add these oils to your diffuser and enjoy.

4. Tangerine Delight Diffuser Recipe

15 Drops of Vanilla Oil

2 Drops of Tangerine Oil

Directions:

Add these oils to your diffuser and enjoy.

5. Orange You Wonderful Diffuser Recipe

10 Drops of Orange Oil

25 Drops of Vanilla Oil

Directions:

Add these oils to your diffuser and enjoy.

6. Wake Up Now Diffuser Recipe

2 Drops of Lemon Oil

2 Drops of Ylang Ylang Oil

1 Drop of Basil Oil

Directions:

Add these oils to your diffuser and enjoy.

7. Rise & Shine Diffuser Recipe

6 Drops of Rosemary Oil

3 Drops of Peppermint Oil

2 Drops of Ginger Oil

2 Drops of Basil Oil

Directions:

Add these oils to your diffuser and enjoy.

8. Vanilla & Citrus Dream Diffuser Recipe

5 Drops of Vanilla Oil

1 Drop of Orange Oil

1 Drop of Tangerine Oil

Directions:

Add these oils to your diffuser and enjoy.

9. Energize Up Diffuser Recipe

2 Drops of Cinnamon Cassia Oil

1 Drop of Rosemary Oil

1 Drop of Peppermint Oil

Directions:

Add these oils to your diffuser and enjoy.

10. Brighter Skies Diffuser Recipe

6 Drops of Tangerine Oil

2 Drops of Lemon Oil

1 Drop of Grapefruit Oil

1 Drop of Lime Oil

Directions:

Add these oils to your diffuser and enjoy.

11. Fruit In The Forest Diffuser Recipe

4 Drops of Bergamot Oil

2 Drops of Cypress Oil

2 Drops of Juniper Berry Oil

Directions:

Add these oils to your diffuser and enjoy.

12. Express & Uplift Diffuser Recipe

10 Drops of Neroli Oil

4 Drops of Tangerine Oil

4 Drops of Ylang Ylang Oil

Directions:

Add these oils to your diffuser and enjoy.

13. Fulfill & Uplift Diffuser Recipe

10 Drops of Bergamot Oil

3 Drops of Lemon Oil

1 Drop of Lime Oil

Directions:

Add these oils to your diffuser and enjoy.

14. Energy Blend Diffuser Recipe

3 Drops of Lemon

3 Drops of Peppermint

3 Drops of Rosemary

Directions:

Add these oils to your diffuser and enjoy.

15. Burst Of Energy Diffuser Recipe

3 Drops of Rosemary

3 Drops of Peppermint

2 Drops of Grapefruit

Directions:

Add these oils to your diffuser and enjoy.

16. Energy Blaster Diffuser Recipe

3 Drops of Frankincense

3 Drops of Wild Orange

2 Drops of Cinnamon

Directions:

Add these oils to your diffuser and enjoy.

17. Wake Up Alert Diffuser Recipe

4 Drops of Peppermint

4 Drops Wild Orange

Directions:

Add these oils to your diffuser and enjoy.

18. Happy Happy Blend Diffuser Recipe

3 Drops of Lavender

3 Drops of Bergamot

2 Drops of Geranium

Directions:

Add these oils to your diffuser and enjoy.

19. Pure Happiness Diffuser Recipe

2 Drops of Lime

2 Drops of Peppermint

2 Drops of Frankincense

2 Drops of Wild Orange

Directions:

Add these oils to your diffuser and enjoy.

20. Get Energized Diffuser Recipe

2 Drops of Cinnamon Oil

2 Drops of Frankincense Oil

2 Drops of Wild Orange Oil

Directions:

Add these oils to your diffuser and enjoy.

21. Fatigue Relief Recipe

1 Tablespoon of Extra Virgin Olive Oil

3 Drops of Ginger Oil

3 Drops of Peppermint Oil

Directions:

Mix all your ingredients together. Massage mixture into areas of your body that are feeling fatigued.

22. Energy Shot Recipe

1 Tablespoon of Jojoba Oil

2 Drops of Roman Chamomile Oil

2 Drops of Sandalwood Oil

Directions:

Mix all your ingredients together. Massage mixture into your chest when you need a boost of energy.

Essential Oils Homemade Aromatic Recipes To Help With Weight Loss

Blending your essential oils together is a wonderful way to experiment using your favorite scents. It allows you to achieve the healing qualities of each of the oils while also creating new helpful blends. The blends in this section will help with dissolving fat and suppressing appetite. These are all easy to make and I suggest trying them out for yourselves to see which ones are right for you. My personal favorites are the Rejuvenating Bath and Craving Curbing Salve, while my wife enjoys the Anti-Cellulite Rub and Fat Reducing Massage.

1. Anti-Cellulite Rub Oil Recipe

10 Drops of Grapefruit Oil

5 Drops of Rosemary Oil

2 Drops of Peppermint Oil

2 Drops of Ginger Oil

2 Drops of Cypress Oil

Directions:

Combine all your drops. Blend with a carrier oil before you apply to your body.

2. Fat Reducing Massage Recipe

1/4 Cup of Almond Oil

5 Drops of Lemon Oil

5 Drops of Grapefruit Oil

5 Drops of Cypress Oil

Directions:

Mix all ingredients together before applying.

3. Appetite Suppressing Diffuser Recipe

40 Drops of Mandarin Oil

20 Drops of Lemon Oil

12 Drops of Ginger Oil

12 Drops of Peppermint Oil

Directions:

Blend together all your drops. Add a few drops of your blend to your diffuser.

4. Rejuvenating Bath Recipe

5 Drops of Grapefruit Oil

5 Drops of Ginger Oil

5 Drops of Sandalwood Oil

5 Drops of Orange Oil

5 Drops of Lemon Oil

Directions:

Add each of these to your warm bath before getting in.

5. Craving Curbing Salve Recipe

1/2 Cup of Olive Oil

80 Drops of Fennel Oil

40 Drops of Bergamot Oil

24 Drops of Patchouli Oil

Directions:

Mix ingredients together. Massage them on your abdomen.

6. Metabolism Boosting Soak Recipe

2 Tablespoons of Jojoba Oil

10 Drops of Cypress Oil

10 Drops of Rosemary Oil

8 Drops of Grapefruit Oil

Directions:

Draw a bath and add all of your ingredients before getting in.

7. Appetite Stimulant Recipe

3 Drops of Lime Oil

3 Drops of Spearmint Oil

2 Drops of Ginger Oil

Directions:

Mix ingredients together. Inhale directly from the bottle. Keep away from your eyes.

8. Weight Loss Citrus Blend Recipe

1 Teaspoon of Coarse Sea Salt

30 Drops of Grapefruit Oil

4 Drops of Lemon Oil

1 Drop of Ylang Ylang Oil

Directions:

Add everything to a small bottle or inhaler and take 3 deep, slow, long breaths. Take a quick break and repeat. Do this three time in total. Sniff hard and long in each nostril. Do this before eating or when your appetite is triggered.

9. Weight Loss Mint Blend Diffuser Recipe

1 Teaspoon of Coarse Sea Salt

20 Drops of Peppermint Oil

10 Drops of Bergamot Oil

4 Drops of Spearmint Oil

1 Drop of Ylang Ylang Oil

Directions:

Add everything to a small bottle or inhaler and take 3 deep, slow, long breaths. Take a quick break and repeat. Do this three time in total. Sniff hard and long in each nostril. Do this before eating or when your appetite is triggered.

10. Weight Loss Herbal Blend Diffuser Recipe

1 Teaspoon of Coarse Sea Salt

15 Drops of Marjoram Oil

15 Drops of Basil Oil

1 Drop of Thyme Oil

1 Drop of Oregano Oil

Directions:

Add everything to a small bottle or inhaler and take 3 deep, slow, long breaths. Take a quick break and repeat. Do this three time in total. Sniff hard and long in each nostril. Do this before eating or when your appetite is triggered.

11. Cellulite Help Recipe

15 ML of Grape Seed Oil

6 Drops of Grapefruit Oil

4 Drops of Lemon Oil

2 Drops of Rosemary Oil

2 Drops of Cypress Oil

Directions:

Mix all your ingredients together and apply topically as needed. Avoid direct sunlight once applied.

12. Cellulite Relief Recipe

1/2 Ounce of Carrier Oil

2 Drops of Chamomile

2 Drops of Cypress Oil

2 Drops of Yarrow Oil

2 Drops of Geranium Oil

Directions:

Mix all your ingredients together and dot on areas as needed.

13. Cellulite Salt Scrub Recipe

1 Cup of Seal Salt

1/2 Cup of Jojoba Oil

7 Drops of Grapefruit Oil

5 Drops of Cypress Oil

3 Drops of Patchouli Oil

Directions:

Mix all your ingredients together and apply topically as needed. Avoid direct sunlight once applied.

14. Crave Reducer Diffuser Recipe

6 Drops of Eucalyptus Oil

Directions:

Add oil to your diffuser to help cut down on cravings. Should use in the rooms where you spend the most amount of your time.

15. Metabolism Increaser Recipe

1 Drop of Ginger Oil

1 Drop of Grapefruit Oil

1 Drop of Peppermint Oil

1 Drop of Lemon Oil

Directions:

Mix all your ingredients together. Add mixture to your first and final drink of each day.

16. Stop Over Eating Recipe

2 Drops of Grapefruit Oil

1 Glass of Water

Directions:.

Add your oil to your glass of water before eating. Do this before each meal.

17. Reduce Sugar Cravings

2 Drops of Roman Chamomile Oil

1 Glass of Water

Directions:.

Add oil to a glass of water before drinking. Do this several times a day.

Essential Oils Mind, Emotional Support & Balance Recipes

In this section, I'm going to go over a few recipes that are good when you need to clear your mind and find more balance or clarity in your life.

1. State of Blissful Thinking Diffuser Recipe

6 Drops of Sandalwood Oil Blend

3 Drops of Orange Oil

3 Drops of Ginger Oil

Directions:

Add these oils to your diffuser and enjoy.

2. Wash Away The Blues Diffuser Recipe

3 Drops of Orange Oil

2 Drops of Lemon Oil

2 Drops of Clove Oil

Directions:

Add these oils to your diffuser and enjoy.

3. Self Reflection Meditation Diffuser Recipe

3 Drops of Patchouli Oil

2 Drops of Clove Oil

1 Drop of Sandalwood Oil Blend

Directions:

Add these oils to your diffuser and enjoy.

4. Male Clarity Diffuser Recipe

5 Drops of Sandalwood Oil Blend

2 Drops of Cypress Oil

1 Drop of Atlas Cedar Oil

Directions:

Add these oils to your diffuser and enjoy.

5. Get Centered Diffuser Recipe

2 Drops of Rose Absolute Oil

2 Drops of Germanium Oil

2 Drops of Clary Sage Oil

Directions:

Add these oils to your diffuser and enjoy.

6. Perfect Harmony Diffuser Recipe

3 Drops of Chamomile Oil

2 Drops of Neroli Oil

2 Drops of White Thyme Oil

2 Drops of Hyssop Oil

2 Drops Of Bergamot Oil

Directions:

Add these oils to your diffuser and enjoy.

7. Flower Meditation Diffuser Recipe

5 Drops of Rose Absolute Oil

1 Drop of Geranium Oil

Directions:

Add these oils to your diffuser and enjoy.

8. Sharper Mental Focus Diffuser Recipe

3 Drops of Eucalyptus Oil

2 Drops of Tangerine Oil

2 Drops of Peppermint Oil

Directions:

Add these oils to your diffuser and enjoy.

9. Head Relief Diffuser Recipe

3 Drops of Lavender Oil

3 Drops of Chamomile Oil

3 Drops of Peppermint Oil

Directions:

Add these oils to your diffuser and enjoy.

10. Study Session Diffuser Recipe

5 Drops of Rosemary Oil

5 Drops of Peppermint Oil

2 Drops of Frankincense Oil Blend

Directions:

Add these oils to your diffuser and enjoy.

11. Keep Calm & Focused Diffuser Recipe

3 Drops of Patchouli Oil

3 Drops of Cedarwood Oil

3 Drops of Lavender Oil

Directions:

Add these oils to your diffuser and enjoy.

12. Rise & Shine Diffuser Recipe

6 Drops of Rosemary Oil

3 Drops of Peppermint Oil

2 Drops of Ginger Oil

2 Drops of Basil Oil

13. Center & Grounding Diffuser Recipe

10 Drops of Sandalwood Oil Blend

5 Drops of Patchouli Oil

3 Drops of Ginger Oil

Directions:

Add these oils to your diffuser and enjoy.

14. Strengthen & Stabilize Diffuser Recipe

10 Drops of Sandalwood Oil Blend

4 Drops of Cedarwood Oil

3 Drops of Ginger Oil

Directions:

Add these oils to your diffuser and enjoy.

15. Mental Clarity Recipe

15 ML of Jojoba Oil

8 Drops of Rosemary Oil

4 Drops of Lemon Oil

4 Drops of Peppermint Oil

Directions:

Mix all your ingredients together and rub in as needed. Avoid direct exposure to sunlight after applying.

16. Emotional Exhaustion Recipe

1 Ounce of Vegetable Oil

7 Drops of Lavender Oil

5 Drops of Hyssop

5 Drops of Grapefruit

Directions:

Mix all your ingredients together and use in a full body massage as needed. Avoid direct exposure to sunlight after applying.

17. Ancestors Essence Recipe

15 ML of Jojoba Oil

8 Drops of Frankincense Oil

8 Drops of Lime Oil

2 Drops of Sandalwood Oil

2 Drops of Patchouli Oil

2 Drops of Opoponax Oil

Directions:

Mix all your ingredients together and apply as needed.

18. Night Bath Blend Recipe

2 Tablespoons of Honey

1 Drop of Lavender Oil

1 Drop of Palmarosa Oil

1 Drop of Chamomile Oil

Directions:

Mix all your oils together and stir in your honey. Add mixture to a warm bath.

19. Shaman's Journey Recipe

15 ML of Marula Oil

4 Drops of Jasmine Oil

2 Drops of Palo Santo Oil

2 Drops of Sandalwood Oil

1 Drop of Cedar Oil

Directions:

Mix all your ingredients together and apply as needed.

20. Palo Santo Purify Bath Recipe

1 Cup of Epsom Salt

2 Drops of Grapefruit Oil

2 Drops of Palo Santo Oil

2 Drop of Palmarosa Oil

2 Drops of Cypress Oil

Directions:

Mix all your ingredients together and add to your bath.

21. A Soothed Mind Diffuser Recipe

7 Drops of Frankincense Oil

6 Drops of Cistus Oil

3 Drops of Sandalwood Oil

Directions:

Add these oils to your diffuser and enjoy.

22. A Meditative Blend Recipe

30 ML of Jojoba Oil

8 Drops of Frankincense Myrrh Oil

6 Drops of Sandalwood Oil

3 Drops of Cedar Oil

3 Drops of Opoponax Oil

Directions:

Mix all your ingredients together and apply as needed.

23. Life Transitioning Recipe

15 ML of Marula Oil

4 Drops of Clary Sage Oil

4 Drops of Fennel Oil

2 Drops of Geranium Oil

1 Drop of Melissa Oil

Directions:

Mix all your ingredients together and apply as needed.

24. Focused Relief Diffuser Recipe

7 Drops of Cypress Oil

5 Drops of Lavender Oil

3 Drops of Grapefruit Oil

2 Drops of Vetiver Oil

2 Drops of Cedar Oil

Directions:

Add these oils to your diffuser and enjoy.

25. Mood Balancer Blend Diffuser Recipe

4 Drops of Clary Sage Oil

4 Drops of Neroli Oil

2 Drops of Jasmine Oil

Directions:

Add these oils to your diffuser and enjoy.

26. Rested Rejuvenation Blend Recipe

15 ML of Jojoba / Rose Hip Oil Blend

8 Drops of Clary Sage Oil

8 Drops of Vetiver Oil

8 Drops of Lavender Oil

Directions:

Mix all your ingredients together and apply as needed.

27. Rested Meditation Blend Recipe

30 ML of Jojoba Oil

8 Drops of Frankincense Oil

6 Drops of Sandalwood Oil

3 Drops of Cedarwood Oil

3 Drops of Frankincense Myrrh Oil

Directions:

Mix all your ingredients together and apply as needed.

28. Gain Focus Diffuser Recipe

2 Drops of Peppermint Oil

2 Drops of Wild Orange Oil

Directions:

Add these oils to your diffuser and enjoy.

29. Breathe Deeply Diffuser Recipe

1 Drop of Ylang Ylang Oil

1 Drop Of Patchouli Oil

1 Drop of Bergamot Oil

Directions:

Add these oils to your diffuser and enjoy.

30. Insomnia Relief Recipe

30 ML of Sweet Almond Oil

10 Drops of Roman Chamomile Oil

5 Drops of Lavender Oil

3 Drops Of Patchouli Oil

2 Drops of Cedarwood Oil

Directions:

Mix all your ingredients together in a dark bottle. Shake well. Massage mixture into skin thoroughly approximately 1 hour before bed.

31. Higher Self Confidence Recipe

3 Drops of Spearmint Oil

1 Blank Inhaler

Directions:

Place oil into your inhaler. Inhale deeply as needed.

32. Self Acceptance Recipe

5 Drops of Jasmine Oil

1 Blank Inhaler

Directions:

Place oil into your inhaler. Inhale deeply as needed.

Essential Oils Love, Romance, & Relationship Recipes

In this section, I'm going to go over a few recipes that are good when you want to fan the flames of love and romance.

1. Botanical Bliss Diffuser Recipe

5 Drops of Rose Absolute Oil

2 Drops of Ylang Ylang Oil

Directions:

Add these oils to your diffuser and enjoy.

2. On Cloud 9 Diffuser Recipe

5 Drops of Patchouli Oil

4 Drops of Sandalwood Oil Blend

1 Drop of Rose Absolute Oil

1 Drop of Ylang Ylang Oil

Directions:

Add these oils to your diffuser and enjoy.

3. Exotic Nights Diffuser Recipe

3 Drops of Orange Oil

2 Drops of Ylang Ylang Oil

Directions:

Add these oils to your diffuser and enjoy.

4. Perfect Passion Diffuser Recipe

6 Drops of Jasmine Absolute Oil

5 Drops of Geranium Oil

Directions:

Add these oils to your diffuser and enjoy.

5. Soft Touch Diffuser Recipe

13 Drops of Jasmine Absolute Oil

1 Drop of Bergamot Oil

1 Drop of Ylang Ylang Oil

Directions:

Add these oils to your diffuser and enjoy.

6. Sweetest Romance Diffuser Recipe

7 Drops of Vanilla Oil

2 Drops of Clary Sage Oil

2 Drops of Cedarwood Oil

1 Drop of Orange Oil

Directions:

Add these oils to your diffuser and enjoy.

7. Feeling Wonderful Diffuser Recipe

15 Drops of Rose Absolute Oil

1 Drop of Geranium Oil

Directions:

Add these oils to your diffuser and enjoy.

8. Love Is Here Diffuser Recipe

5 Drops of Geranium Oil

3 Drops of Jasmine Absolute Oil

1 Drop of Patchouli Oil

Directions:

Add these oils to your diffuser and enjoy.

9. Feeling Sweet Diffuser Recipe

2 Drops of Chamomile Oil

2 Drops of Ylang Ylang Oil

Directions:

Add these oils to your diffuser and enjoy.

10. Sweet Cinnamon Diffuser Recipe

6 Drops of Tangerine Oil

4 Drops of Cinnamon Cassia Oil

2 Drops of Nutmeg Oil

Directions:

Add these oils to your diffuser and enjoy.

11. Romance Blend Recipe

15 ML of Marula Oil

4 Drops of Sandalwood Oil

4 Drops of Jasmine Oil

2 Drops of Cardamom Oil

2 Drops of Rose Oil

Directions:

Mix all your ingredients together and apply topically.

12. Romantic Nectar Love Potion Recipe

55 Drops of Orange Oil

41 Drops of Mandarin Oil

19 Drops of Sandalwood Oil

13 Drops of Vanilla Absolute Oil

11 Drops of Cardamom Oil

8 Drops of Ginger Oil

8 Drops of White Ginger Lily

7 Drops of Jasmine Absolute Oil

4 Drops of Patchouli Oil

Directions:

Mix all your ingredients together and apply topically. Avoid exposure to direct sunlight after application.

13. Love Potion Blend Recipe

40 Drops of Sandalwood Oil

31 Drops of Vanilla Absolute Oil

20 Drops of Orange Oil

18 Drops of Neroli Oil

16 Drops of Mandarin Oil

12 Drops of Jasmine Oil

11 Drops of Cardamom

11 Drops of Grapefruit Oil

10 Drops of Saffron Attar Oil

8 Drops of Vetiver Oil

8 Drops of Blue Lotus Oil

8 Drops of Fir Oil

4 Drops of Marigold Oil

Directions:

Mix all your ingredients together and apply topically. Avoid exposure to direct sunlight after application.

14. Smooth Love Potion Recipe

36 Drops of Ylang Ylang Oil

30 Drops of Rose Geranium Oil

15 Drops of Melissa Oil

13 Drops of Rose Absolute Oil

11 Drops of Ginger Oil

10 Drops of Zdravetz Oil

5 Drops of Cinnamon Oil

Directions:

Mix all your ingredients together and apply topically. Avoid exposure to direct sunlight after application.

Essential Oils Recipes For The Home

In this section, I'm going to go over a few recipes that are good for around the house. I use many of these on a weekly basis.

1. Cleaning Assist Mist Cleaner Spray Recipe

12 Drops of Tea Tree Oil

12 Drops of Eucalyptus Oil

12 Drops of Pinon Pine Oil

8 Drops of Grapefruit Oil

Directions:

Mix all your ingredients together in an 8-ounce mist bottle. Avoid direct exposure to sunlight.

2. Room Deodorizer Diffuser Recipe

8 Drops of Silver Fir Oil

4 Drops of Cypress Oil

4 Drops of Juniper Oil

4 Drops of Cedarwood Oil

Directions:

Add these oils to your diffuser and enjoy.

3. Deodorizer Room Spray Recipe

2 Cups of Water

6 Drops of Lemon Oil

6 Drops of Tea Tree Oil

3 Drops of Cedarwood Oil

3 Drops of Clove Oil

1 Drop of Cinnamon Oil

Directions:

Mix all your ingredients together in a spray bottle. Avoid direct exposure to sunlight.

4. Mosquito Breeding Spray Recipe

2 Cups of Water

Squirt Of Dish Washing Soap

1/2 Ounce of Neem Oil

10 Drops of Eucalyptus Oil

5 Drops of Catnip Oil

Directions:

Mix all your ingredients together in a spray bottle. Shake and squirt wherever mosquitoes breed.

5. Liquid Soap Recipe

4 Ounces of Castille Soap

8 Drops of Rhododendron Oil

8 Drops of Sweet Orange Oil

2 Drops of Cedarwood Oil

1 Drop of Ginger Oil

Directions:

Mix all your ingredients together and shake well before using.

6. Mosquito & Bug Spray Recipe

4 Ounces of Distilled Water

8 Drops of Palo Santo Oil

8 Drops of Eucalyptus Oil

8 Drops of Lemongrass Oil

4 Drops of Pinon Pine Oil

4 Drops of Peppermint Oil

Directions:

Mix all your ingredients together in a spray bottle. Shake and spray to soothe bites and repel bugs.

7. Garden Insect Spray Recipe

4 Drops of Sweet Orange Oil

2 Drops of Roman Chamomile Oil

2 Drops of Lavender Oil

2 Drops of Grapefruit Oil

Directions:

Mix all your ingredients together in an 4-ounce bottle. Spray the affected leaves. Avoid direct exposure to sunlight if you get any on your skin.

8. Say Goodbye Insect Blend Diffuser Recipe

4 Drops of Citronella Oil

4 Drops of Peppermint Oil

4 Drops of Spearmint Oil

1 Drop of Lemongrass Oil

Directions:

Add these oils to your diffuser and say goodbye to insects.

9. Insect Begone Diffuser Recipe

2 Drops of Thyme Oil

2 Drops of Basil Oil

2 Drops of Eucalyptus Oil

2 Drops of Lemon Grass Oil

Directions:

Add these oils to your diffuser and say goodbye to insects.

10. Insect Repellent Diffuser Recipe

1 Drop of Melaleuca Oil

1 Drop of Lemon Grass Oil

1 Drop of Rosemary Oil

1 Drop of Eucalyptus Oil

1 Drop of Thyme Oil

Directions:

Add these oils to your diffuser and say goodbye to insects.

11. Bugs Begone! Diffuser Recipe

1 Drop of Eucalyptus Oil

1 Drop of Thyme Oil

1 Drop of Lemongrass Oil

1 Drop of Basil Oil

Directions:

Add these oils to your diffuser and say goodbye to insects.

12. Farewell Odor Diffuser Recipe

2 Drops of Lemon Oil

1 Drop of Lime Oil

1 Drop of Cilantro Oil

1 Drop of Melaleuca Oil

Directions:

Add these oils to your diffuser and enjoy a cleaner smelling home.

13. All Purpose Cleaner Recipe

3 Drops of Eucalyptus Oil

2 Drops of Rosemary Oil

Directions:

Mix all your ingredients together and add to a bottle 3/4 filled with water. Spray on areas as needed.

14. Anti-Microbial Recipe

1 Tablespoon of Jojoba Oil

3 Drops of Rosemary Oil

2 Drops of Lemongrass Oil

1 Drop of Thyme Oil

Directions:

Mix all your ingredients together and apply to surfaces in your home that need cleaning.

15. Floor Cleaner Recipe

1 Quart of Water

1/4 Cup of Distilled White Vinegar

3 Drops of Eucalyptus Oil

2 Drops of Lemongrass Oil

Directions:

Mix your water and white vinegar together. Add the essential oils. Apply to your floor using a mop. Rinse with clean water after applied for a few minutes.

16. Laundry Recipe

25 Drops of Eucalyptus Oil

Laundry Detergent

Directions:

Add your oil to your laundry detergent and shake well to mix together. Use on clothes.

17. Pet Dander Diffuser Recipe

3 Drops of Peppermint Oil

2 Drops of Ginger Oil

1 Drop of Thyme Oil

Directions:

Add these oils to your diffuser. Use as needed in rooms frequented by your pets.

18. Beat Stains Recipe

2 Drops of Lemongrass Oil

Directions:

Rub your oil onto your stain and allow to set for a few minutes. Place in your washing machine.

19. Window Cleaner Recipe

1 Cup of White Vinegar

10 Drops of Lemon Oil

Water

Directions:

Add your water and white vinegar to a spray bottle until it is 3/4 of the way full. Shake it well to combine. Add the lemon oil and shake again to combine. Spray on any windows that need cleaning and wipe off with your paper towel.

20. Litter Box Cleaner Recipe

1 Cup of White Vinegar

2 Drops of Lavender Oil

Directions:

Use vinegar while cleaning the litter box. Then dilute your lavender in a bottle of water. Rinse your litter box out with this water mixture.

Essential Oils Recipes For Your Pets

In this section, I'm going to go over a few recipes that are good for treating your pets. I hope they help you as much as they have me over the years. Remember to always do your research on an oil before using it on your pets or yourself. Don't put the safety of your pet at risk because you didn't take the time beforehand to do your due diligence. Using essential oils on your pet inappropriately could lead to side effects including death.

1. Calming Your Pet Recipe

1 Tablespoon of Jojoba Oil

6 Drops of Valerian Oil

4 Drops of Lavender Oil

4 Drops of Bergamot Oil

4 Drops of Sweet Marjoram Oil

2 Drops of Roman Chamomile Oil

Directions:

Mix all your ingredients together. Rub 4 drops between your hands and apply to your pet's ears, between their thighs, and under their armpits.

2. Improve Eyesight Recipe

15 ML of Sweet Almond Oil

4 Drops of Frankincense Oil

2 Drops of Cypress Oil

2 Drops of Rosemary Oil

Directions:

Mix all your ingredients together. Massage mixture onto the back and chest of your pets.

3. Pet Shampoo Recipe

8 Ounces of All Natural Shampoo

10 Drops of Geranium Oil

8 Drops of Rose Oil

8 Drops of Petitgrain Oil

5 Drops of Ylang Ylang Oil

Directions:

Mix all your ingredients together. Apply to your pet and wash off.

4. Sinus Infection Recipe

20 ML of Sweet Almond Oil

10 Drops of Eucalyptus Oil

8 Drops of Ravensara Oil

6 Drops of Myrrh Oil

Directions:

Mix all your ingredients together. Massage mixture onto the neck and chest of your pets.

5. Flea Treatment Recipe

1 Tablespoon of Olive Oil

10 Drops of Peppermint Oil

6 Drops of Clary Sage Oil

6 Drops of Lemon Oil

4 Drops of Citronella Oil

Directions:

Mix all your ingredients together. Apply the mixture to the neck, back, legs, tail, and chest of your pets.

6. Congestion Treatment Diffuser Recipe

15 ML Sweet Almond Oil

5 Drops of Ravensara Oil

5 Drops of Myrrh Oil

5 Drops of Eucalyptus Oil

Directions:

Mix all your ingredients together and add to your nebulizing diffuser. Must be given to your pets 4 times a day for 5 to 10 minutes per time as needed.

7. Teething Pain Remedy Recipe

20 ML of Sweet Almond Oil

20 Drops of Clove Bud Infusion Oil

6 Drops of Myrrh Oil

4 Drops of Roman Chamomile Oil

Directions:

Mix all your ingredients together. Place a few drops on a frozen soft toy and give to your pet so they can chew and relieve their pain as they're playing.

8. Immunity Booster Recipe

15 ML of Sweet Almond Oil

2 Drops of Thyme Oil

2 Drops of Bay Laurel Oil

2 Drops of Eucalyptus Oil

2 Drops of Niaouli Oil

2 Drops of Coriander Seed Oil

2 Drops of Ravensara Oil

Directions:

Mix all your ingredients together. Massage mixture into the back and chest of your pet.

9. Skin Allergy Recipe

20 ML of Sweet Almond Oil

10 Drops of Lavender Oil

6 Drops of Chamomile Oil

5 Drops of Geranium Oil

2 Drops of Carrot Seed Oil

Directions:

Mix all your ingredients together. Rub 4 drops between your hands and apply to your pet's ears, between their thighs, and under their armpits.

10. Tick Repellent Remedy Recipe

60 Drops of Olive Oil

1 Drop of Lavender Oil

Directions:

Mix your ingredients together. Pour a couple drops on the tick and allow it to sit for a little bit. Extract the tick and wipe away any excess oil.

11. Combat Rheum Recipe

2 Drops of Eucalyptus Oil

Hot Water

Directions:

Mix your ingredients together. Allow your pet breathe in the steam. Be sure to keep your pet from burning themselves on the water.

12. Defeat Motion Sickness Recipe

20 ML of Jojoba Oil

12 Drops of Peppermint Oil

8 Drops of Ginger Oil

Directions:

Mix your ingredients together. Apply mixture to your pet's ears, thighs, coat, and armpits.

13. Repel Mosquitoes Recipe

10 Ounces of Aloe Vera Juice

30 Drops of Citronella Oil

12 Drops of Myrrh Oil

12 Drops of Rose Geranium Oil

12 Drops of Lemongrass Oil

Directions:

Mix your ingredients together in a spray bottle. Spray over your pet's coat. Avoid the eyes.

14. Fresh Smelling Breath Recipe

20 ML of Sweet Almond Oil

10 Drops of Cardamom Oil

8 Drops of Coriander Seed Oil

6 Drops of Peppermint Oil

Directions:

Mix your ingredients together in a small sized glass bottle. Use a dropper and give your pets 3 drops every day to improve their breath.

15. Reduce Anxiety Recipe

20 ML of Sweet Almond Oil

8 Drops of Petitgrain Oil

6 Drops of Bergamot Oil

2 Drops of Ylang Ylang Oil

2 Drops of Sweet Basil Oil

1 Drop of Neroli Oil

Directions:

Mix your ingredients together. Massage a small amount onto the chest of your pet as needed.

16. Dry Paws Recipe

70 Drops of Coconut Oil

1 Drop of Lavender Oil

Directions:

Mix your ingredients together. Place on your pet's pads using a cotton pad. Can also put in special socks to keep them from getting at the mixture.

17. Nice Coat Remedy Recipe

4 Drops of Rosemary Oil

2 Drops of Grapefruit Seed Oil

All Natural Shampoo

Directions:

Mix your ingredients together. Apply shampoo to pet and wash them with water.

18. Arthritis Remedy Recipe

15 ML of Jojoba Oil

6 Drops of Rosemary Oil

4 Drops of Ginger Oil

3 Drops of Lavender Oil

Directions:

Mix your ingredients together. Massage mixture onto your pet's sore joints.

Conclusion

Thanks for reading my book. I hope this guide on essential oils has provided you with all the information you needed to get going. Don't put off getting started. The sooner you begin, the sooner you'll start to notice an improvement in your health and well-being. While results may vary, they will come if you stick to the information found in this book.

Remember that not all essential oils are created equal. Always get the highest quality oils you can afford. Be sure to follow all directions and safety precautions when using your essential oils. Be extra attention when using these items on children, pets, or pregnant women. It may take some time to build yourself a good collection of essential oils but over time you'll begin to figure out which oils you prefer and tend to use on a consistent basis.

I hope you enjoyed all the essential oil recipes I've included in this book. There's no shortage of recipes to try out. Feel free to experiment and create your own. I suggest sticking to these recipes in the beginning while you're still learning and developing your essential oils knowledge base. If you still have any unanswered questions I suggest checking out one of the resource sites or apps I discussed earlier. When I first got started learning about essential oils these sites had all the answers I needed. They were truly an invaluable resource to have at my disposal.

Good luck. I wish you nothing but the best!

Made in the USA
San Bernardino, CA
08 November 2016